QUALITY AND SAFETY IN ANAESTHESIA

QUALITY AND SAFETY IN ANAESTHESIA

Edited by
J SECKER WALKER
Senior Lecturer, University College London Medical School;
Medical Adviser, Quality and Risk Management Ltd,
Merrett Health Risk Management Ltd

BMJ
Publishing
Group

© BMJ Publishing Group 1994

First published in 1994 by the BMJ Publishing Group, BMA House, Tavistock Square, London WC1H 9JR

British Library Cataloguing in Publication Data
A catalogue record for this book is available from the British Library

ISBN 0 7279 0828 6

The following picture sources are acknowledged: Chapter 10, fig 2, with permission, Gravenstein JS, *Gas monitoring and pulse oximetry*, 1990, Butterworth-Heinemann. Chapter 10, fig 3, Copyright Universal Press Syndicate, with kind permission. The chapter *Psychology and Safety in Aviation* is British © Crown Copyright 1993/MOD: published with the permission of the Controller of Her Brittanic Majesty's Stationery Office.

Typeset, printed and bound in Great Britain by Latimer Trend & Company Ltd, Plymouth

Contents

CONTENTS

Foreword

Major reforms in the NHS have included increasing involvement in "quality" issues. I recognise, of course, that some of these reflect a worldwide movement. To the novice the structured as opposed to the intuitive pursuit of quality may seem excessively contrived and cynics can enjoy a field day. With time, however, the sense of it becomes better understood and enthusiasm may follow. The guidance and authority of this work will, I hope, do much to ensure that the pursuit of quality is achieved effectively and efficiently.

If, as I believe, this book is devoted to the science of quality then the reader must understand, as I am sure the authors do, that it is all at an embryonic level. Nevertheless, Kelvin's aphorism about measurement and understanding should not be forgotten. Neither should Florence Nightingale's, which can be paraphrased as "good management assures quality at all times and not just at optimal times."

Is quality free? Some say so, but I have found no sign of it. As I write, much time is being drained from potential direct service to patients to set the infrastructure for "quality" in the future. Whether we consider the risk manager, the nurse manager (quality), or the clinical director of the department of anaesthesia, there needs to be accountability for these innovations. There may even be a day of reckoning. There would be quality in that, too.

November 1993   ALASTAIR A SPENCE
                                        President, Royal College of Anaesthetists

Preface

The original title for this book was *Audit and Anaesthesia*, yet medical audit is really only a means to an end, the end being the provision of a service to the patient that is both safe and of the highest quality. The chapters that follow suggest how medical audit can be used to monitor and improve agreed standards and also explore facets of anaesthetic practice that help ensure safety for the patient.

Most anaesthetic accidents are caused at least in part by human error and while good design of equipment and routine monitoring is of great importance, an attempt to understand the reasons why individual anaesthetists make mistakes seems to be worthwhile. Training and continuing education are essential parts of the anaesthetic process and in future the speciality is likely to use simulators to prepare trainees for dealing with potential disasters. In addition, like many big companies, the speciality may perhaps consider what type of psychological profile trainee anaesthetists should possess.

I thank the authors for the quality of their product and for delivering their chapters so promptly and Mary Banks and the *BMJ* team for all their advice and support.

March 1994   J SECKER WALKER

1 Quality and the management of risk

J SECKER WALKER

The motto of the Association of Anaesthetists, "In somno securi-tas" (safety in sleep) is the assumption that all patients make as they drift into unconsciousness and the outcome that anaesthetists strive to achieve. Our continual attempts to monitor and improve anaesthetic practice are directly related to our ability to provide safe anaesthesia. The word quality, nowadays commonly used in the NHS, is difficult to define, describes an abstract idea, and is interpreted differently by different people. It has, however, a close association with what we perceive to be an "acceptable standard." Improvement in quality can be gained by agreeing standards that are superior to those currently "acceptable" and then achieving those standards.

Ideas about the setting of standards and the measurement of the efficacy of medical care date back to the early part of this century with the work of Hey Groves in the United Kingdom[1] and Ernest Amory Codman in the United States.[2] A review of their ideas together with the minimum standards set by the American College of Surgeons was published in 1924,[3] and shows the modern clinician that the profession is not treading unknown paths but rather has new information technology for the collection and analysis of data which assist with the definition of current perform-ance and aid the setting of future standards. The main aims of medical audit are to set standards, and to monitor and improve the quality of medical care. At the same time it should be an educa-tional activity and indicate areas where patient care can be deli-vered more efficiently. Efficiency inevitably involves the cost of care whether in terms of time, staff, or money. In an environment

1

in which cash is limited one profligate doctor deprives another doctor's patients of the resources for medical care.

Medical practice can be considered in terms of the structure, process, and outcome of medical care.[4]

The *structure* is the organisation within which we practise, be that the trust, the unit, the department or the operating theatre. There are areas here in which we may attempt to set standards to alter our working or educational environment for the better so that patient care and safety improves and staff are encouraged to function to the best of their ability.

The *process* of medical care is the area that receives most attention when quality and audit are discussed, because it focuses on the interaction between doctor and patient and is the easiest to understand. Most organisational data are collected about process and so there are more things to measure and so more standards to set. The news about discrepancies in the histopathological examination of specimens of bone tumours in Birmingham brings home to clinicians the value of properly conducted medical audit in maintaining appropriate standards.[5]

The *outcome* of care is the most difficult to measure although it is the most often discussed. In anaesthesia outcome is perhaps easier to measure as most patients recover from anaesthesia without serious side effects, mortality is low, and major complications are rare. Various methods of auditing anaesthetics have been discussed ranging from review of notes; mortality and morbidity meetings; exception, complication, and critical incident reporting; and reviews of postgraduate education and adherence to departmental protocols and standards of equipment.[6]

Risk management and total quality management

High quality anaesthesia should be free of risk, and the management of risk is an important part of medical audit. Since medical defence organisations withdrew from NHS hospitals there has been a need to manage risk in the United Kingdom, and several companies are already in the market to provide risk analysis and management techniques.

Increasing numbers of big organisations are adopting "total quality management" (TQM) as their fundamental philosophy. TQM has been defined as "the process of conscious and continued striving on the part of all staff to attain zero defects in all aspects of the organisation's activities." Looked at this way, the Japanese idea of "kaizen" – every defect is something to be learned from – becomes eminently sensible, for only by identifying defects can one rectify them and follow the path to total quality.[7] Accidents that occur to patients are definitely "defects," whether they are accidents or the result of negligence. In either case, methods of managing the risk of their occurrence should be a part of any quality management programme. In the NHS Review White Paper, the Department of Health defined medical audit as "the systematic critical analysis of the quality of medical care, including the procedures used for diagnosis and treatment, the use of resources, and the resulting outcome and quality of life for the patient."[8] Medical audit, clinical audit, and risk management are therefore all part of our progress towards total quality, together with efficient administration and financial probity.

"Risk management" is a term that covers all aspects of an organisation's activity and can apply to the risks associated with property management or investment as well as to the effect of the poor performance of employees or malfunctioning equipment. In this chapter I will deal with the risk management that relates to dealing with the results of adverse events to patients and the implementation of programmes to prevent accidents happening.

A four year analysis of the relationship between medical injury, negligence, costs, compensation and lawsuits in the United States produced interesting results.[9 10] After reviewing 30 121 sets of casenotes, a total of 3·7% of patients admitted to hospital were found to have sustained injuries that resulted in measurable disability. Drug complications were the most common (19%) followed by wound infection (14%) and technical complications (13%). Of all the adverse events reported, 48% were associated with an operation and 28% were the result of negligence, but surgical adverse events were less likely to be the result of negligence than non-surgical events. The percentage of adverse events resulting from negligence was considerably higher among elderly patients. Of the patients injured, 57% recovered completely within a month, and 70% recovered within six months. Half of the 14% of fatal injuries were the result of negligence. The authors found that the total number of malpractice claims was 10% of the number of negligent injuries, but only 2% of the patients reported to have had a negligent injury actually filed a claim. They suggested that of the 3·7% of patients in hospital who have an adverse event, 1% are the

3

result of negligence. A similar large study in California reported rates of 4·6% and 0·8%, respectively.[11] If one were to assume that British hospitals are no safer, a hospital with 25 000 inpatients/year could expect about 250 negligent adverse events/year.

The rising costs of subscriptions in the United Kingdom to defence organisations and the proposed introduction of differential rates depending on specialty (which would be reflected in the doctors pay review recommendations) caused the government to appraise three options for the future. The first was to make no changes and to accept that pay rises should reflect rising defence subscriptions; the second was that health authorities should take on all new liabilities; and the third option, which was the one chosen, was to take on new and contingent liabilities from 1 January 1990 with a contribution of about £50 million from the defence organisations' reserves. Until that date the medical defence organisations had stood the cost of adverse medical litigation and had handled the claims, so the experience of handling such risks in provider units was relatively meagre. The history in the USA has been quite different; plaintiffs have sued both hospital and doctor ("going for the biggest pocket") and so risk management programmes are well established.

Risk management in hospitals

What is a risk? Each of us takes risks every day and each of us would define the level of risk for a certain activity in a different way from each other. Risk management has been defined by Runciman as: the cost effective reduction of risk to levels perceived to be acceptable to society.[12]

Risks can be divided into three main groups: those that have a direct impact on patient care (for example, a disconnected ventilator), those that have an indirect impact on patient care (for example, loss of power supply or lack of clean instruments), and health and safety risks (for example, sharps injuries). The four stages of assessment and management of risk are: to identify what can go wrong, to measure how often it goes wrong, to put controls in place to prevent it going wrong again, and to find money to pay for losses if it does go wrong.

To supervise this, each hospital should have a particular officer responsible for the risk management programme, who is closely integrated with medical audit or quality assurance. This relationship is logical, because adverse events that affect patients obviously have a quality component. There are two complementary parts of the job of the risk manager: to deal with claims (either real or potential), and to prevent damage to patients or staff occurring in the first place. The outstanding requirement in both is an organisational will to reduce risk backed by a continuing and updated educational programme. In addition, early communication with, and explanation to, patients when an adverse event has occurred is an essential means of reducing the likelihood of subsequent litigation. The box lists the ways in which a claim may be identified.

Ways in which a claim is identified

- Report of an incident
- Report of a complaint
- Request for access to patient's records by patient or lawyer
- Information from patient's representative
- Verbal or telephone information from doctor or nurse involved in accident
- Analysis of patient satisfaction surveys

Incident reporting

Incident reporting is essential in the recognition and prevention of risks and managerial drive is needed to ensure that employees understand its importance and use. To report an actual or potential incident on an "incident form" must be accepted as a normal part of everyday life and should not be used as part of a disciplinary process. Medical audit databases can be used to indicate areas of potential risk, such as an unexpected return to theatre or an unscheduled admission to the intensive care unit. Other information from such systems may indicate whether operating at night is appropriate and being done by the correct grade of surgeon, whether the operations done are as listed, and whether the patient's notes were available. Entry of data from incident reports and complaints permits a picture to be built up of where the potential risks in the organisation are, and it should indicate areas that would benefit from review of working practices and protocols.

5

Dealing with complaints

Investigation and handling of complaints are important areas in which litigation may be prevented by correct action. The risk manager should be kept fully informed about complaints and their progress, and a database can indicate the types of complaint by specialty, or by consultant, or by site. Patterns of complaint may emerge to show where management time should be spent now to avert risks in the future.

Analysis of patient satisfaction surveys provides useful insight into where patients think the hospital is failing, and customised patient surveys of departments that accrue more complaints than expected can be a useful investigative tool.

The medical records department and doctors should be aware of the importance of informing the risk manager whenever a patient or lawyer requests access to hospital records. The notes should be reviewed with the doctor, nurse, and representative of the patient, and cross checked against the database of incidents to discover as early as possible whether there may be any substance to a subsequent claim.

Protection against hazards

The risk manager must be known to be responsible for ensuring that patients and staff are as free from hazards as possible, for protecting the organisation against litigation, and for looking after the interests of employees who are faced with a claim against their professional handling of a case. If the risk manager is seen to support staff, doctors and nurses will be motivated to report untoward events when they occur. The concept of "early warning" of a clinical accident should be part of the fundamental philosophy of a risk management programme.[13] Adverse events should be reported as soon as possible after they have occurred, which will allow the risk manager to assemble relevant facts systematically and quickly while recall is fresh, to identify the relevant medical and other records that must be retained as material evidence, and to allow staff to communicate rapidly and truthfully with the patient before anger "at not being told the truth" sets in with the inevitable determination to seek redress in the courts. In addition, a cultural change is required so that staff become aware of and report areas of potential danger to themselves and the patients (for example, disposal of sharps) using the incident reporting procedure. Managers can then put matters right before someone is injured.

Communication with patients

Part of the educational programme should be aimed at persuading staff to communicate fully with patients at all times and particularly after an adverse event. This does not mean admitting negligence, merely that an adverse event has taken place and that staff will do all in their power to help. Part of this process of communication relates to the issue of informed consent by which patients are made aware of the risks that their treatment may entail.

The importance of good communication with patients cannot be overestimated. Data about complaints in University College London Hospitals during the past two years indicate consistently that many complaints from patients are about lack of communication and courtesy. Many American hospitals employ a "patient representative" whose job it is to meet the patient on admission and keep in touch thereafter to answer questions about the care the patient is receiving or the working of the hospital, and to listen to suggestions as to how to improve the service. The patient representative is informed of any adverse event that occurs to that patient, and will immediately visit the patient and talk about the problem. At the same time the representative will liaise with the risk manager to attempt to reduce the chance of a claim being filed.

The risk manager will therefore be in a position to identify areas of risk to patients and employees, which will allow clinical directors and managers to run educational programmes and put protocols for working practice in place that will reduce the likelihood of accidents. Organisations such as the Medical Defence Union and lawyers used to dealing with medical litigation have much useful data which can be used to identify the most vulnerable points in each specialty.

Risk management in anaesthesia

Mortality associated with anaesthesia alone was reported to be about 1/10 000 by Lunn and Mushin,[14] 3/10 000 by Tiret,[15] and the Confidential Enquiry into Perioperative Deaths (CEPOD) reported that only three deaths out of nearly half a million resulted from anaesthesia alone (see chapter 10).[16] The role of major

7

complications in anaesthesia is variously reported as 0·45% by Cohen et al in a review of 112 000 anaesthetics[17] and 0·13% by Tiret et al in a prospective study of 198 103 anaesthetics in France.[15]

Perception of risk

The problem with risks in anaesthesia concerns the psychology of the perception of risk. Patients understand that operations are inherently dangerous, but though they know that anaesthetic accidents do happen occasionally, they feel that they should not. The possibility of surgical failure seems to be accepted by both patient and surgeon, whereas the anaesthetist enjoys no such luxury and anaesthetic failure is all too often assumed to be negligent.

Despite the perception of many patients that anaesthesia is safe, the anaesthetist does what is potentially extremely dangerous. Patients are deprived of most protective reflexes by unconsciousness; they may be paralysed; given a mixture of different gases to breathe and doses of potentially toxic drugs; they may have major physiological interventions with induced hypotension, intentional or unintentional hypothermia, and altered clotting mechanisms; and they may rely entirely on mechanical devices to ventilate them and circulate their blood. What the public expects to be a safe adjunct to operation, therefore, is actually inherently dangerous and so the latitude and understanding that anaesthetists can expect from a damaged patient is slight.

Databases

An important part of any risk management programme is the ability to collect and analyse data, and medical audit databases in anaesthesia should be able to provide such data about the operative course of all patients. In addition, these systems should be able to show where the process is failing – for example, picking up complications, critical incidents, and administrative failures such as missing notes or a change in the order of the operating list. Regular analysis of such data will identify where attention should be focused to reduce risk.

According to Utting, the most common complaint to the Medical Defence Union was of damage to teeth which made up 52% of reports,[18] but Aitkenhead (Lecture to Royal College of Anaesthetists Continuing Medical Education Day, Royal Society of

Medicine, October 1992) listed the pattern of more serious injuries that lead to actual or threatened litigation. Table I breaks down the 150 claims between 1989 and 1990.

TABLE I   Causes of 150 claims made to Medical Defence Union about adverse events during anaesthesia 1989–90.

Cause	Percentage
Brain or spinal cord damage	24
Postoperative death	17
Awareness during general anaesthesia	12
Death during anaesthesia	12
Pain during regional anaesthesia	8
Peripheral nerve damage	4
Fetal death	1
Suxamethonium pains	1
Miscellaneous injuries including fractured ribs, tissued infusion sites, pneumothorax, and laryngeal damage	21

Of the deaths and cases of brain damage, no less than 48% occurred postoperatively. In their prospective study Tiret et al showed that 42% of major complications occurred in the postoperative period.[15] Gannon reviewed 25 anaesthetic deaths that were reported to the Medical Protection Society between 1982 and 1986 (table II).[19]

TABLE II   Causes of 22 anaesthetic deaths reported to the Medical Protection Society 1982–6.

Cause	Number
Failed intubation	10
Drug related (overdose or sensitivity)	6
Malfunction of equipment	4
Total spinal anaesthesia and failure to intubate	2

Malfunction of the equipment included incorrect assembly of the anaesthetic system, failure of the ventilator, and disconnection. Utting et al, over a decade earlier, had reviewed 326 cases of death or brain damage during anaesthesia that had been reported to the Medical Defence Union, half of which were thought to be the result of "faulty technique"; of these two thirds concerned hypoxia, or problems with the airway or ventilator.[20] Both Lunn and Mushin[14] and the report of CEPOD[16] showed that failure to apply knowledge was an important factor in three quarters of

9

anaesthetic deaths, and Cooper *et al* showed that 82% of preventable incidents resulted from human error and only 14% from failure of equipment but poor design of equipment was partially involved with many of the human errors.[21] Interestingly, there were strong indications that injuries associated with anaesthesia, like aircraft accidents, did not usually result from isolated errors. Rather, they resulted from a combination of errors that taken together caused circumstances in which the anaesthetist failed to identify the problem. A later paper by Cooper *et al* listed the 10 most common critical incidents, of which 70% were related to failure to ventilate the lungs with oxygen (table III).[22]

Other factors associated with anaesthetic mortality and morbidity have been consistently reported by various authors.[5 6 10 12–14 17] These include inadequate supervision of junior staff, lack of proper preoperative assessment, failure to carry out equipment checks, failure of communication, poor anaesthetic organisation, poor resuscitation technique, and the absence of the anaesthetist from the operating theatre. This last may now lead to a charge of manslaughter. Two anaesthetists have been found guilty of manslaughter since 1990. Any risk management programme, therefore, must review the various aspects of the anaesthetic service (box).

Monitoring

It is of course the cases of cerebral or spinal cord damage that cause the most expensive litigation. Brain damage stems from failure to deliver oxygen to the brain for one of three reasons: failure of the oxygen supply, failure of the delivery of oxygen to the lungs, and failure of transport of oxygen from the lungs to the

TABLE III   Incidence of 10 most common "critical incidents" in anaesthetic complaints.

Incident	Percentage of reports
Disconnection of breathing circuit	27
Inadequate gas flow	22
Syringe swap	19
Problems with gas supply	15
Disconnected intravenous line	11
Malfunction of laryngoscope	11
Premature extubation	10
Misconnection of circuit	9
Hypovolaemia	9
Problem with endotracheal tube	7

Aspects of the anaesthetic service that must be reviewed as part of risk management

- Monitoring
- Medical records
- Communication and informed consent
- Checks of equipment
- Procedures in the operating theatre
- Supervision of junior staff
- Staffing and procedures in the recovery room
- Continuing medical education
- Critical incident analysis (chapter 7)

---

brain. The hazards that pose most risk to the patient are gas mixtures and flows, gas circuits, tracheal intubation, and ventilation. This is therefore a sensible starting point for attempting to reduce risk. The awards obtained by litigation for brain damage have increased considerably, as has the sophistication of anaesthetic machines and monitors. Human error will always be a feature of accidents, but there is now evidence that if minimum standards of monitoring are complied with, the number of anaesthetic accidents will be reduced.[23] Tinker et al reviewed 1175 anaesthetic related malpractice claims between 1974 and 1988,[24] of which there was sufficient information available in 1097 for the reviewers to make a judgement. Nearly a third of the negative outcomes would have been prevented by additional monitors, and these cases were the worst rated. The monitors that the reviewers regarded as the most useful were pulse oximetry and pulse capnometry.

Expecting an anaesthetist to work without monitors is like expecting a pilot to fly an airliner without any instruments or warning devices. Over the past few years (since the adoption of minimal standards in the United States) the cost of malpractice claims against anaesthesiologists has decreased by about two thirds and in the Harvard group of hospitals in Boston insurance premiums for anaesthesiologists have been reduced by 40%.[25] In 1991 the annual insurance premium for the Risk Management Foundation of the Harvard Medical Institutions for a staff anaesthesiologist was $11 750, for a urologist $15 980, for a gynaecologist $28 200, and for an obstetrician or orthopaedic surgeon $35 250.

If minimum standards of monitoring are implemented, the risk of hypoxic injury will be considerably lessened because the anaesthetist will have been alerted to trouble early enough to do something about it. Of all the developments in monitoring that have been introduced during the last decade, the pulse oximeter is probably the most cost effective. Because many are portable they can be used in the anaesthetic room and the recovery area as well as in the operating theatre. There are also devices that will sound an alarm when the ventilator becomes disconnected from the endotracheal tube. These alarms may cost less than £500, and there is no excuse in cost-benefit terms for not using them. Meters that show the concentration of inspired oxygen will warn when the concentration of oxygen in the inspired mixture falls below a safe level before the pulse oximeter registers the problem and are especially valuable in "circle" systems. Capnography, especially when the carbon dioxide tension is shown graphically, is of great help in describing the pattern of ventilation to the anaesthetist and it also indicates clearly whether the endotracheal tube is positioned correctly. The more modern the anaesthetic machine the more likely it is to have a device that prevents nitrous oxide being given in concentrations that will cause hypoxia; indeed, the newer machines have many of the above devices built in, including blood pressure monitors and electrocardiograms. Such machines cost £25 000 or more, but Aitkenhead estimated that discounted over a 10 year period such a machine would add £4 to the cost of each operation.[26] This is a tiny proportion of the total cost, and it will not only help prevent accidents, reduce litigation, and improve quality, but also it will release current monitors for use in anaesthetic rooms and particularly in recovery areas (where we must remember about half the cases of death and cerebral damage occur).

Medical records

The next area for attention in reducing the risk of litigation is the maintenance of good anaesthetic records. It is not well known that if the plaintiff receives legal aid, the hospital is likely to have to pay its own costs after a court case even if it wins the case, and this may be as much as £100 000. If the anaesthetic records are properly kept the expert witness for the plaintiff will have much less chance of alleging that it is probable that the cause of brain damage was a hypoxic episode, in the absence of evidence to the contrary. The case may well then be settled out of court.

Complete monitoring systems have been developed that allow continuous printouts of physiological data and the anaesthetist can mark drugs and events on the same chart. These printouts provide valuable evidence as to exactly what took place and when. It is important, however, to note clearly if the monitors should give misleading readings for whatever reason.

Communication and informed consent

Good communication with patients is one of the most effective means of preventing litigation if something goes wrong, and for the anaesthetist this communication must start with the preoperative visit. Gannon indicated that inadequate preoperative assessment, including history taking, was a causative factor in 28% of anaesthetic deaths studied.[19] Patients now expect to give "informed" consent to the procedures carried out.

Lord Justice Bridge stated in his judgement in the case of Sidaway v Bethlem Royal Hospital Governors and others in the House of Lords: "When specifically questioned by a patient of apparently sound mind about risks involved in a particular treatment proposed, a doctor's duty must, in my opinion, be to answer both truthfully and as fully as the questioner requires". Lord Scarman in a minority judgement said that the doctor should be liable "where the risk is such that in the court's view a prudent person in the patient's situation would have regarded it as significant."

The current legal position is that the decision as to how much discussion of risks is best calculated to help a patient to make a rational choice about whether to undergo a particular treatment must be a matter of clinical judgement.[28] Clinical judgement, however, is subject to the definitive test for the duty of care owed by medical practitioners as propounded in the Bolam case: "whether or not the doctor had acted in accordance with the practice accepted as proper by a body of responsible and skilled medical opinion even though other doctors adopted a different practice."[29]

It is sensible to warn patients about the possibility of damage to teeth, because over half the anaesthetic complaints to the Medical

Defence Union before 1990 related to this. If regional anaesthesia is proposed the possibility of pain or discomfort (7·5% of claims) should be discussed, and the patient should be told what action the anaesthetist would then take; if the patient is clearly unhappy at the prospect and there is no strong contraindication for general anaesthesia, it would probably be wiser to opt for the latter. If general anaesthesia and regional anaesthesia are to be used, it is sensible to explain this to the patient (or next of kin). An entry reporting the preoperative visit and the issues discussed should be made in the patient's notes.

Checks of equipment

Many authors have emphasised that failure to check equipment and drugs is one of the most common of human failures in anaesthetic misadventures.[22 30–32] Lunn and Mushin reported that the anaesthetic machine had not been tested before use in 17·8% of the cases they reported. The anaesthetist is always held responsible for the functioning of the equipment he or she uses and for the drugs given. Aspects that should be monitored particularly carefully are the labelling of syringes, "do it yourself" repairs to equipment, allowing other staff to draw up drugs, and checking that the vaporiser is actually full.

Procedures in the operating theatre

Each operating theatre should have strict procedures for checking the patient, the intended operation, and the signature on the consent form. The operating list should have clearly displayed the patients' names, hospital numbers, and intended operations, and the order in which they will be done. It should be altered only for emergencies, and all patients should be accompanied by their notes and results of laboratory investigations. Anaesthetic audit databases should be used to monitor the administrative aspects of the patient's progress through the operating theatre and recovery room. Most North American patient incident reports show that the operating theatre is potentially the most dangerous place in the hospital and this is borne out by the survey of Brennan et al[6] who found that 48% of all adverse events were associated with an operation. Unpublished data from University of London hospitals' anaesthetic database show that between 10% and 15% of all visits

14

to the operating theatre are associated with one or more "administrative errors." Theatres that have a consistently high level of administrative errors can be identified and appropriate action taken. Good operating theatre procedures ensure that patients are appropriately positioned and are protected against injury to eyes, nerves, and skin, and against diathermy burns.

Supervision of junior staff

Lack of supervision of junior anaesthetists is a consistent factor in anaesthetic accidents. Both Lunn and Mushin[14] and the report of CEPOD[16] commented that operative mortality is to some degree related to the supervision of trainees in anaesthesia, particularly when patients are very sick, elderly, or being operated on as emergency cases. Cooper *et al* reported that lack of supervision was the most common factor in anaesthetic mishaps, while Gannon stated that inadequate supervision was a factor in 32% of the anaesthetic deaths that he studied.[19] Clinical directors of departments of anaesthesia are responsible for ensuring that the service provided for each list is given by appropriately qualified anaesthetists and that junior staff are aware of guidelines and rules, particularly when they should call for assistance. The report of CEPOD recommended that a consultant should be responsible for all elective lists and said that it was "rubbish" to state that no one was responsible for what trainees do.[16] That report is a public document and its recommendations are well known to the lawyers of plaintiffs, so it behoves clinicians to have good reasons if they do not follow them. Medical audit databases provide excellent information about the degree of supervision and types of cases that juniors are undertaking and, together with data on complications and critical incidents, provide useful insights into where risk can be reduced – for instance, by reorganising consultants' sessions.

Staffing and procedures in the recovery room

The introduction of recovery rooms, provided that they are appropriately staffed and equipped, should lead to a reduction in the number of accidents that occur in the immediate postoperative period. The return to a surgical ward where the degree of supervision is necessarily much less, however, places sick patients at risk and the anaesthetist may be criticised for sanctioning discharge to the ward too soon. There is also the danger of an anaesthetic error causing postoperative difficulties; for example, progressive respiratory failure could be linked by a plaintiff's counsel with aspiration during the operation. The 24 hour "post-anaesthetic recovery" rooms in which patients stay after serious operations in many American hospitals have much to commend them. They also have the advantage that because an anaesthetic trainee is always present, proper pain relief can be maintained and accurate records of postoperative complications kept.

Continuing medical education

The importance of postgraduate education and training has been emphasised by many of the articles about adverse events in anaesthesia. Anaesthetists sometimes liken themselves to airline pilots who have to be recertified regularly throughout their careers to keep their licences. It cannot be long before consultant anaesthetists have to attend continuing medical education courses regularly.

It is interesting to speculate how NHS hospital trusts will learn to cope with the risks of litigation. Whether or not they are allowed to insure, there will be a powerful incentive to keep legal costs as low as possible because these will have to be added to prices which in turn may reduce competitiveness. During the next few years the trusts may start to take a more active role in requiring their doctors to follow patterns of treatment that the trust board considers to be safest. This is a considerable departure from the commonly held view that the consultant alone decides the course of treatment that the patient will undergo. An example of this in anaesthesia would be that anaesthetists were allowed to induce hypotension deliberately only in defined circumstances. It is also likely that trusts will no longer give tenure when appointing consultants but offer a three or five year rolling contract. As in North America, renewal of the consultant's contract may depend on evidence of continuing medical education and an acceptable amount of litigation.

1 Hey Groves EW. Surgical statistics: a plea for a uniform registration of operation results. *BMJ* 1908;ii:1008–9.
2 Roberts JS, Coale JG, Redman RR. A history of the Joint Commission on Accreditation of Hospitals. *JAMA* 1987;258:936–40.
3 American College of Surgeons. The minimum standard. *Bulletin of the American College of Surgeons* 1924;8:1–4.

4 Donabedian A. Evaluating the quality of medical care. *Millbank Memorial Federation of Quality* 1966;**2**:166–203.
5 Rayment T, Lightfoot E, Rogers L. Cancer fiasco: the lost eight years. *The Sunday Times* 1993 Aug 29; 2 (col 6).
6 Secker-Walker J. Audit in anaesthesia. In: Kaufman L, ed. *Anaesthesia Review 8*. Edinburgh: Churchill Livingstone, 1991.
7 Ellwood PM. Shattuck Lecture – outcomes measurement. *N Engl J Med 1988*;**318**:1549–56.
8 Department of Health. *Working for patients*. London: HMSO, 1989.
9 Brennan TA, Leape LL, Laird NM, Herbert L, Localio AR, Lawthers AG, *et al.* Incidence of adverse events and negligence in hospitalized patients – results of the Harvard Medical Practice Study 1. *N Engl J Med* 1991;**324**:370–7.
10 Leape LL, Brennan TA, Laird NM, Lawthers AG, Localis AR, Barnes BA, *et al.* The nature of adverse events in hospitalized patients – results of the Harvard Medical Practice Study 2. *N Engl J Med* 1991;**324**:377–84.
11 California Medical Association. *Report of the Medical Insurance Feasibility Study*. San Francisco: California Medical Association, 1977.
12 Runciman WB. Risk assessment in the formulation of anaesthesia safety standards. *Eur J Anaesthesiol* 1993;**10**(Suppl 7):26–32.
13 Lindgren OH, Christensen R, Harper Mills D. Medical malpractice risk management early warning systems. *Law and Contemporary Problems* 1991;**54**:23–41.
14 Lunn JN, Mushin WW. *Mortality associated with anaesthesia*. London: Nuffield Provincial Hospitals Trust, 1982.
15 Tiret L, Desmonts J-M, Hatton F, Vourc'h G, *et al.* Complications associated with anaesthesia – a prospective survey in France. *Canadian Anaesthetists Society Journal* 1986;**33**:336–44.
16 Buck N, Devlin HB, Lunn JN. *Report of a Confidential Enquiry into Perioperative Deaths (CEPOD)*. London: Nuffield Provincial Hospitals Trust/King's Fund, 1987.
17 Cohen MH, Duncan PG, Pope WDB, Wolkenstein C, *et al.* A survey of 112,000 anaesthetics at one teaching hospital. *Canadian Anaesthetists Society Journal* 1986;**33**:22–31.
18 Utting JE. Pitfalls in anaesthetic practice. *Br J Anaesth* 1987;**59**:877–90.
19 Gannon K. Mortality associated with anaesthesia. *Anaesthesia* 1991;**46**:962–6.
20 Utting JE, Gray TC, Shelley FC. Human misadventure in anaesthesia. *Canadian Anaesthetists Society Journal* 1979;**26**:472–8.
21 Cooper JB, Newbower RS, Long CD, McPeek B. Preventable anesthesia mishaps. *Anesthesiology* 1978;**49**:399–406.
22 Cooper JB, Newbower RS, Kitz RJ. An analysis of major errors and equipment failure in anesthesia management: considerations for prevention and detection. *Anesthesiology* 1984;**60**:34–42.
23 Eichhorn JH. Prevention of intraoperative anesthesia accidents and related severe injury through safety monitoring. *Anesthesiology* 1989;**70**:572–7.
24 Tinker JH, Dull DL, Caplan RA, Ward RJ, Cheney FW. Review of 1175 anesthesia related malpractice claims between 1974 and 1988. *Anesthesiology* 1989;**71**:541–6.
25 Taylor TH, Goldhill DR. Standards and Audit. In: *Standards of Care in Anaesthesia*. Oxford: Butterworth-Heinemann, 1992.
26 Aitkenhead AR. *Risk management in anaesthesia*. Healthcare Risk Management Bulletin No 2. London: Medical Defence Union Publications, 1992.
27 Sidaway v Bethlem Royal Hospital Governors and others [1985] 2 WLR 480.
28 Brazier M. *Medicine, patients and the law*. 2nd ed. London: Penguin Books Ltd, 1992:73–93.
29 Bolam v Friern Hospital Management Committee [1957] 1 WLR 582, 587–8.
30 Craig J, Wilson ME. A study of anaesthetic misadventures. *Anaesthesia* 1981;**36**:933–6.
31 Cundy J, Baldock GJ. Safety check procedures to eliminate faults in anaesthetic machines. *Anaesthesia* 1982;**37**:161–9.
32 Ward CS. *Anaesthetic equipment*. 2nd ed. London: Baillière Tindall, 1985.

2 National quality studies in anaesthesia

JOHN N LUNN

"Quality is that characteristic of an activity that can be improved."[1] This aphorism encapsulates my view of the topic of this book. An organisation or culture may wish to implement change but this ambition is unproductive unless there is also improvement. But improvement from what? Bedrock information about the state of affairs in advance of any change is almost essential so that subsequent developments can be assessed in relation to supposed and assumed improvements. If this baseline control is missing or unreliable it is likely that demonstration of positive change will be impossible.

This chapter traces the development of national studies of the practice of anaesthesia.

Evolution

The Association of Anaesthetists of Great Britain and Ireland met this problem some years ago when it wished to acquire data about the safety of the then current practice of anaesthesia so as to have a basis on which to gauge any deterioration. (Yes, deterioration; it was at a time of serious medicopolitical stress). This requirement was used in the submission for funds to support the study which culminated in the report *Mortality Associated with Anaesthesia*.[2] The acknowledged aim of that study was to determine the incidence of death in 1979 in order to be able to compare similar rates in the future. Absence of denominator data in the Association's previous enquiries (1956 and 1960) had rendered them less valuable for this purpose. Somewhat limited agreement was obtained with our surgical colleagues. The often quoted rate of one death, within six days after 10 000 operations totally as a result of anaesthesia, was confirmed in the folklore of anaesthesia. There were many other results of this enquiry but the fundamental aim was realised and a figure for deaths associated with anaesthesia in the United Kingdom was established.

The next realisation was that conclusions about the practice of anaesthesia based on what was done for patients who subsequently died might not represent ordinary normal practice—that is, the sample might be skewed. This naturally led to the question, what is the paradigm (general pattern or example) of the practice of anaesthesia in the United Kingdom? This was an entirely new problem and one which had not received any significant attention in the United Kingdom before. Once again the Association of Anaesthetists started things off, this time with their *Survey of Anaesthetic Practice (SOAP)*.[3] This was originally planned for 1983 but was finally completed in 1987. It was a formidable undertaking whereby volunteer anaesthetists of all grades were invited to complete quite extensive questionnaires about 25 successive anaesthetics for which they were responsible. Surprisingly more than 400 anaesthetists complied with this request and data on 10 666 anaesthetics were collected from all over the country.

The report of this survey was not published formally because doubts were expressed about the validity of some of the data. Such was the anxiety about confidentiality that anonymity was absolute and it was impossible to verify some items which were questionable. "Nevertheless there is a substantial amount of information which is of legitimate interest to anaesthetists," and, it should be noted, this information is not available anywhere else. Three developments happened as direct consequences of SOAP. Working parties were established by the Association to consider monitoring during anaesthesia and tests of anaesthetic machines before use, and the publications which followed had considerable impact on the practice of anaesthesia.[45] It was then considered desirable for these matters to be handled in the future by the then College of Anaesthetists which established a quality of practice unit. One of the first actions of this unit was to conduct another enquiry by questionnaire into the incidence of cardiac arrest and brain damage. The findings of the latter were not published formally (but are available from the Royal College of Anaesthetists).

Temporary cardiac arrest was confirmed to be less uncommon than some might have hitherto assumed.

Substantial changes in obstetric anaesthesia have occurred in the United Kingdom since the inception of the *Confidential Enquiry into Maternal Deaths*, which started more than 40 years ago. The triennial reports indicate quite clearly that avoidable events during anaesthesia that cause death have declined to an almost irreducible level. Denominator data of interest to anaesthetists (numbers of caesarean sections under epidural anaesthesia and under general anaesthesia) are now retrieved and thus it is to be hoped that regular comparisons will be possible in the future.

This Enquiry is a national cooperative one among obstetricians, pathologists, and anaesthetists, and its multispecialty composition influenced the development of the *Confidential Enquiry into Perioperative Deaths (CEPOD)* and also the recently announced *Confidential Enquiry into Stillbirths and Deaths in Infancy (CESDI)*. These enquiries are unusual features of medicine in the United Kingdom and are not duplicated anywhere else in the world. All manner of developments in medicine happen simultaneously and it is not realistic to assume that all improvements in outcome are solely the result of confidential enquiries. It is probable nevertheless that the attention which is drawn by their reports to deficiencies in clinical management does have significant effect.

Interim period

The outstanding deficiency in the anaesthetist-led study mentioned above was the absence of significant involvement of surgeons. This was also the case with all the other studies in the world, which, although they pay lip-service to the ideal of surgical enmeshment with these matters, have also failed to include them realistically.[67] One or two fortuitous events combined to stimulate the Association of Anaesthetists to approach the Association of Surgeons of Great Britain and Ireland with the result that, after protracted negotiations with numerous organisations, CEPOD was established. This was independent of all individual specialties, overseen by a steering committee (representative of all specialties), and funded by two charities (The Nuffield Provincial Hospitals Trust and King's Fund for London). An enquiry was started (which subsequently was appreciated effectively to be a pilot for a national one) in three regions of the National Health Service in

England (Northern, South Western, and North East Thames). The enquiry revealed the high standard of anaesthesia and surgery which was achieved in the regions at that time. The overall crude death rate of 0·7% within 30 days of a surgical procedure is an acceptable figure and compares well with figures from elsewhere. There were some differences in clinical management, the amount of consultant supervision, and out of specialty operating between the three regions studied.

The recommendations of this Enquiry were first published in 1987 and since they remain relevant are reproduced below.[8]

Quality assurance

(1) There is a need for an assessment of clinical practice on a national basis. Our experience suggests that our colleagues would welcome this.

(2) Consultants in every district should ensure that their own coding and input to information systems (including the Korner systems) is accurate and up to date; without this, any audit is flawed. Every district should urgently review the storage, movement, and retrieval of patients' notes, particularly those of deceased patients.

(3) Clinicians need to assess themselves regularly. Effective self assessment needs time; time to attend autopsies, mortality/morbidity meetings and clinical review with other disciplines.

Accountability

(4) All departments of anaesthetics and surgery should review their arrangements for consultants' supervision of trainees. Locally agreed guidelines are important to ensure appropriate care of all patients, but particularly when responsibility is transferred from one clinical team, or shift, to another. No senior house officer or registrar should undertake any anaesthetic or surgical operation as an emergency or urgent matter without consultation with their consultant.

Clinical decision making

(5) Resuscitation, assessment and management of medical disease take time and may determine the outcome; their importance needs to be restated. Agreements which permit this in every case are important.

(6) The decision to operate on the elderly and the very sick is important and should be taken at consultant (or senior registrar) level. For the most seriously ill patients, consultant anaesthetists and surgeons should consult together before the operation.

(7) The decision not to operate is difficult. Humanity suggests that patients who are terminally ill or moribund should not have operations (ie non life saving), but should be allowed to die in peace with dignity.

Organisational issues

(8) Districts should review their facilities for out-of-hours work and concentrate anaesthetic, surgical and nursing resources at a single location. A fully staffed and fully equipped anaesthetic room, resuscitation room, operating room, recovery area, and high dependency or intensive therapy unit should be available at all times.

(9) The implementation of the CEPOD classification of operations (emergency, urgent, scheduled, and elective) would concentrate the attention of all staff on the fact that very few operations need to be performed at night.

(10) Operations should only be performed by consultants or junior surgeons (accountable to consultants) who have had adequate training in the specialty relevant to the operation. Health Authorities should therefore balance surgical specialties so that appropriate urological and vascular trained surgeons are provided in each district. In the case of small districts this may necessitate sub-regional units to ensure adequate sub-specialty care. Neurological and neonatal surgery should be carried out at regional units.

When these recommendations are reviewed today it is obvious both how much and how little has changed since that report was published.

Current studies

The maturation of these studies, which is described above, was accompanied by a number of other developments in medicine, surgery, technology, not to exclude anaesthesia itself. These changes have all contributed to the appreciation that anaesthesia is very uncommonly the sole cause of death. Thus the pursuit of changes in rates of death attributable to such a rare cause is likely to be unrewarding. Small errors in the detection of uncommon events have effects on incidence rates which are out of proportion to their magnitude. The opportunity for misinterpretation is too great.

Another change has occurred which is fundamental to the current national enquiries. The early studies concentrated on causation. Peer review of cases was used to determine this to attribute responsibility. It was inherent in this approach that extremes of opinion, benign or malignant, would be expressed. Terms such as "avoidability" or "culpability" or even "assessments" may unnecessarily encourage a sense of guilt in practitioners. Such a response on their part is undesirable, unintended, and probably counterproductive. National CEPOD does not seek to determine *causation* of death but merely uses the occurrence of death as a sampling technique whereby a patient's case is obtained for detailed study. National CEPOD tries to uncover issues of the *quality* in the delivery of anaesthesia and surgery which need to be considered by the public, their politicians, and medical practitioners alike. The linkage between anaesthesia and surgery is essential if the roles of the two specialties are to be clarified.

The protocol for the enquiry states that brief data on all deaths within 30 days of a surgical operation will be collected by National CEPOD. Each year a different sample is chosen for detailed study and a report published. The first year's sample was deaths of children aged less than 10 years of age and in 1990 a random sample (20%) of all deaths was taken.

Role of local audit

The national enquiries have demonstrated the scope for improvement in the delivery of care. Written guidelines for the practice of both surgery and anaesthesia can now be prepared because they can be based on what is known to happen in many places. Agreement between anaesthetists should be easily achieved. Guidelines already exist in many places—for example, for the management of rare events such as anaphylaxis or malignant hyperpyrexia. These are welcomed by most anaesthetists and particularly by trainees who can implement them while they await the arrival of more senior staff, who also may find the advice useful. Ninety per cent of patients are visited by an anaesthetist before operation; there is therefore no hindrance to this criterion becoming a guideline to quality. Eighty nine per cent of the patients who died after operation were monitored during their anaesthetics with a pulse oximeter[9]: this also could easily be implemented as a guideline for standard practice. Such guidelines may start as local ones. They will need to be tested, that is to say, audited. (A financial auditor compares accounts against published and recognised standards of accounting practice.) This process is almost axiomatic to quality. A guideline is designed, written, agreed, promulgated and then actual practice is compared against the guideline. Most efficacious audit processes are those which start with individual enthusiasm and local initiative. Local changes in

23

clinical and organisational management can be readily implemented and then these changes influence national practice and attitudes.

Records

A fundamental, if not the fundamental, part of the pursuit of quality in anaesthesia is to know what has happened at some time in the past in order for comparisons to be made with current practices. This must involve the creation and maintenance of a system of anaesthetic records. Problems of completion of records have always deterred all but the most determined[10]; many frustrations and objections have had to be overcome. The advent of the "new technology" has not solved all of the difficulties, and claims that computers are essential to the practice of audit are not justified; paper and pencil can be used effectively but the effort required may seem to be excessive.

There are residual difficulties with any manual system. The tendency to put a gloss upon events is a well recognised human frailty. This is manifest in anaesthetists no less than others and is exposed clearly.[11 12] Automation of records would, with some reservations, avoid this hazard.

Cooperation and participation

There are always a few individuals who do not wish to contribute to what their peers tell them is "the common good." Much of this reluctance is natural, understandable and is often amenable to change, provided it is based on logical thought. Reservations (the condoms of good ideas) should not be dismissed out of hand; experience shows that there may be some reasonable basis for unease. The hard core of non-participators with National CEPOD is now quite small. (Four consultant anaesthetists.) Laziness is not an acceptable excuse. Individuals can and do still fail to take part in individual cases. National CEPOD has only about 70% cooperation (return of questionnaires) rate despite a 99% acceptance or agree to participate rate. It was less essential to have 100% response rate in studies of causation. Calculated death rates cannot be lower than that determined but may of course be greater. The current cooperation rate by anaesthetists is acceptable and the conclusions are valid although it is obvious that a higher return rate would be preferable and when the sample is random this is even more important.

A different approach to quality assurance is to acquire data about similar operations which had different outcomes, perhaps survival, in order for comparisons to be made. This means that more data must be recovered and this may provoke antipathy or misunderstanding in anaesthetists unless the purpose is clearly understood. The aim is to seek evidence about differences, if any, between the management of patients who die and those who survive. ("You never ask about the many patients who have survived this anaesthetic and operation at my hands.")

National CEPOD has tried two tactics towards this end. Neither were particularly successful. *Survivor* cases were to be patients matched by age, gender, and mode of admission (but from another region than that for the reported death): this method of case control proved absolutely unachievable and was abandoned after the 1989 report. *Index* cases were the first patients who were anaesthetised and operated on by the same team on, or after, a particular date. The returns from this tactic were better but unfortunately the first case was frequently somewhat trivial compared to the patients who died: this method is now not used.

The most recent report dealt with deaths after 15 specific operations.[13] Attention was drawn to the unsolved problem of the prophylaxis against pulmonary thromboembolism, the risks to the elderly of intravenous fluid overload, and the need to match surgical and anaesthetic skills to the state of the patient. The absence of the essential services (24 hour availability of an emergency operating room; recovery rooms; high dependency units; intensive care units) was again criticised, as was the practice of allowing junior trainees of both disciplines to work unsupervised. Important issues for debate among managers, surgeons, and anaesthetists were also suggested.

Facilitation of change and feedback

It is almost fundamental to this type of exercise that the participants should be informed of, not only the results, but also the conclusions of their endeavours. It is important that everyone realises that National CEPOD is the servant, and not the master, of this professional enterprise. *Feedback* is the jargon word. National CEPOD publishes reports. These reports are of anonymous data which initially are sensitive. Bitter early experience suggested that it would be preferable to publish-for-all, public and profession, at the same instant rather than *preferentially* to the medical profession. The data belong to the professions—but it is very important (vital?!) to the public. Changes in this aspect of the protocol, which are designed to mollify the medical profession, are underway.

It is very important for everyone, including anaesthetists, to understand that the Enquiries discussed in this chapter represent a professional attempt at improvement. This is the essence of a profession. The investment of money, effort, and time is not inconsiderable and it behoves us all to take note of and act upon the findings of our Enquiries where appropriate.

1 Imai M. *Kaizen: the key to Japan's competitive success.* New York: Random House, 1986:1–23.
2 Lunn JN, Mushin WW. *Mortality associated with anaesthesia.* London: Nuffield Provincial Hospitals Trust, 1982.
3 *Survey of anaesthetic practice.* London: Association of Anaesthetists of Great Britain and Ireland, 1988.
4 *Recommendations for standards of monitoring during anaesthesia and recovery.* London: Association of Anaesthetists of Great Britain and Ireland, 1988.
5 *Checklist for anaesthetic machines.* London: Association of Anaesthetists of Great Britain and Ireland, 1990.
6 Warden JC, Lunn JN. The role of anaesthesia in death. In: *Baillière's Clinical Anaesthesiology; The anaesthetic crisis.* London: Baillière Tindall, 1993.
7 Forrest JB, Rehder K, Goldsmith CH, *et al.* Multicenter study of general anesthesia. I. Design and patient demography. *Anesthesiology* 1990;72:252–7.
8 Buck N, Devlin HB, Lunn JN. *Report of a confidential enquiry into perioperative deaths.* London: King's Fund and Nuffield Provincial Hospitals Trust, 1987.
9 Campling EA, Devlin HB, Hoile R, Lunn JN. *National confidential enquiry into perioperative deaths (1990).* London: NCEPOD (35 Lincoln's Inn Fields, WC2A 3PN), 1992.
10 Mushin WW, Campbell H, Ng WS. The pattern of anaesthesia in a general hospital. *Br J Anaesth* 1967;39:323.
11 Galletly DC, Rowe WL, Henderson RS. The anaesthetic record; A confidential survey of data omission or modification. *Anaesth Intensive Care* 1991;19:74–8.
12 Rowe WL, Galletly DC, Henderson RS. Accuracy of text entries within a manually compiled anaesthesia record. *Br J Anaesth* 1992;68:381–7.
13 Campling EA, Devlin HB, Hoile R, Lunn JN. *National confidential enquiry into perioperative deaths (1991–2).* London: NCEPOD (35 Lincoln's Inn Fields, WC2A 3PN), 1993.

The reports of NCEPOD may be obtained on application to the address given above.

3 Standards and postgraduate training

ANTHONY P ADAMS

The objectives of training of anaesthetists have been carefully considered by various bodies, most recently by the European Academy of Anaesthesiology, which has published both an overview[1] and a detailed and structured list of procedures in which trainees should become proficient.[2] The letter is based on work that originated from the Australian and New Zealand College of Anaesthetists in 1976 and was updated in 1992.[3] The success of training can be assessed in behavioural terms. Trained people behave more appropriately in all relevant professional circumstances.

This behaviour is of four kinds. Firstly, they have more relevant information immediately available. In educational jargon, they have greater *cognitive* skills. Put simply, they *know more*, and can show this by answering questions in a way that satisfies another trained person. Performance becomes more effective. Secondly, they possess the relevant motor skills: practical performance becomes more effective. Thirdly, they have the ability to make reasoned judgements and implement decisions based on their knowledge and skills, and lastly, instinctive beliefs and attitudes are relevant. The educationalist would say that such anaesthetists have affective skills.

Effective training seeks to develop *all three* of these aspects of behaviour but only the *cognitive* element (and to some extent the attitudes) can be tested by postgraduate examinations such as the Diploma of the Royal College of Anaesthetists and the European Diploma in Anaesthesiology and Intensive Care. *Motor skills* are best assessed during training. *Attitudes* tend to be influenced a lot

27

by the training environment and this is one reason why a satisfactory overall assessment system is needed.

Throughout training, trainees and teachers alike need to be able to assess progress in the acquisition of relevant knowledge and in the attainment of practical motor and judgemental skills and appropriate attitudes. Trainees are often uncertain about what to learn and teachers themselves are not wholly in agreement. One difficulty is the nature of the specialty, which has advanced in many different directions as the skills of the anaesthetist have been applied to many types of patient care. There are difficulties in attempting to define the required content of training. An examination-oriented syllabus easily becomes outdated because it discourages the active search for knowledge outside what has been specified, decreases interest in clinical learning, and impedes the acquisition of skills outside what is actually mentioned.

To meet these difficulties the requisite skills must be set out in the form of learning objectives. In addition to particular subjects learning should automatically include general features (box 1).

Box 1 – General topics that a trainee should learn

- *Clinical experience:* this is most important because, as well as developing manual dexterity and reinforcing knowledge, it contributes to the development of diagnostic and problem solving skills and it fosters the acquisition of attitudes appropriate to the role of a specialist consultant. Appropriate source material such as books, monographs, references, tapes, films, tutorials, and lectures which are relevant to any of the objectives
- *Basic sciences:* it is essential that trainees study the related basic sciences, including pharmacology, physiology, mathematics, and physics
- *General attitude:* trainees should *want to learn* and *want to acquire* practical skills to the best of their ability with the patient's welfare foremost in their minds. The person who wants to train as an anaesthetist must become, above all, a *safe anaesthetist*
- *General features:* even when not stated, all objectives apply to all patients, taking into account age (from the premature infant to the elderly), sex, and genetic make-up
- *Attitude:* is extremely important. Successful learning is substantially dependent on the student's own efforts, so the use of objectives should be the foundation of continuing education and re-education throughout the anaesthetist's professional life

---

Overall aims in the training of anaesthetists

The anaesthetist's skills reflect those qualities which are important in relation to personal attributes, his or her management of patients and relationships with other doctors, members of the health care team, and the community as a whole. The aims of a trainee are shown in box 2.

Training is achieved in several ways: clinical training, academic courses, personal study, and through investigation and research. The small group tutorial system is particularly valuable but seems to be a "British" approach which is regarded as a luxury elsewhere. The assessment of training is made by regular periodic review by senior anaesthetists (in-service assessment), through examinations and through audiovisual material. This includes attendance at and participation in meetings, presenting clinical cases, and publica-

---

Box 2 – Aims of trainees in anaesthetics

- Regard the patient's welfare as pre-eminent
- Become a safe, competent, practical anaesthetist
- Acquire such knowledge, practical skills and attitudes applicable to anaesthesia, analgesia, and intensive care as will most effectively promote the health of the community
- Become competent in those aspects of medicine, surgery, paediatrics, obstetrics, intensive care and other disciplines which are relevant to the practice of a specialist anaesthetist. In turn, trainees should contribute their developing skills as a specialist to these disciplines
- Assign priorities to clinical problems and the resources for the management of these problems in the interests of the patients, their relatives and the community
- Be able to act appropriately as a member or leader of a therapeutic team
- Develop good judgmental skills
- Be willing and able to continue their own education and contribute to the education of nursing, medical, and paramedical staff. Be eager to enquire into clinical and scientific problems, adopting a critical attitude to available information
- Seek to recognise those changes in the specialty, medicine, or society which should modify their practice, and adapt skills accordingly
- Adopt a critical attitude to their own practice and participate in peer reviews of practice and medical audit

tion in scientific journals. The general education of the specialist anaesthetist extends to include the management of clinical services, financial resources, assessment of personnel, and research activities. The final aim is to produce first class anaesthetists who are respected for their clinical skills in the specialty together with the other attributes mentioned above, plus the ability to teach and organise. They should in turn be committed to the welfare and training of younger anaesthetists who follow. All anaesthetists must keep themselves informed of developments in the specialty.

Training requirements for junior staff

Standards are important in any discipline and are absolutely essential in a specialty such as anaesthesia which is at the "sharp end". The reasons why mistakes are made and patients injured during operation and anaesthesia may be the result of a fundamental lack of knowledge or, more often, the failure to apply that knowledge. The formative years are firstly, those of undergraduate medical education when motivation to acquire medical knowledge is nurtured and, hopefully, vocation is strengthened; the preregistration year when young doctors assume a great deal of personal responsibility for patients and when they are likely to start thinking of a choice of future career; and finally, the years of training in the specialty through basic specialist training (formerly known as general professional training) and eventually through higher specialist training (previously called higher professional training). Throughout this time it is the enthusiasm of and example set by seniors (consultants) that inculcates a proper sense of dedication and commitment of care to the patient. Indeed, anaesthetists may be responsible for delaying or rescheduling an operation when they find that the patient is not in an optimal state to have one, and that more can be done to improve the patient's condition and thus make the outcome safer. It is difficult and unfair to blame a junior for taking risks and cutting corners when the example set him by his seniors is poor. Although a consultant may, arguably, justify "cutting corners", his junior knows no better and naturally tends to emulate his chief. A programme of continuing medical education for consultants should therefore have a beneficial effect.

Education must be an integral part of all health service activities.[4] The good education of doctors in the specialty of anaesthesia is the main justification for training posts and is also the best guarantee of continuing high standards and safe practice. The objectives are shown in box 3.[5]

In the nineteenth century mortality resulting from anaesthesia with chloroform, usually given by an open drop method, was probably of the order of 1/2000 patients.[6] Anaesthesia has come a long way since then but it is still a young specialty. In developed parts of the world it has a good safety record although accidents still happen. The importance of the need for education in safety has been emphasised by Norman.[7] In June 1992 at the 10th World Congress of Anaesthesiologists held at the Hague, The World Federation of Societies of Anaesthesiologists adopted the set of international standards for the safe practice of anaesthesia which was developed by *The International Task Force on Anaesthesia Safety*.[8] The general standards of training are summarised in box 4.

Basic specialist training

This period of training leads to the acquisition by examination of the Diploma of Fellow of the Royal College of Anaesthetists (FRCA) or Fellow of the Faculty of Anaesthetists of the Royal College of Surgeons in Ireland (FFARCS Ire). Traditionally this time comprises a year spent as a senior house officer plus the two years as a registrar, making a total of three years training, but many anaesthetists take far more time to complete this stage. Indeed, many senior house officers spend a year in a district general hospital followed by a further year in a teaching hospital or elsewhere before embarking on two or three years of registrar training. There is concern that some aspects of training are

---

Box 3 – Objectives of training in practice

- Gain knowledge and experience in the management of patients undergoing operation including preoperative and postoperative care, intensive care, resuscitation, and pain control
- Gain a thorough grounding in the scientific basis of the practice of anaesthesia
- Develop critical faculties and awareness of the methods and means of research and development in the specialty
- Learn to manage service requirements and to educate the next generation

---

Box 4 – Internationally accepted standards

- *Professional organisations:* anaesthetists should form appropriate organisations at local, regional, and national levels for the setting of standards of practice, supervision of training, and continuing education with appropriate certification and accreditation and general promotion of anaesthesia as an independent professional specialty
- *Training, certification, and accreditation:* adequate time and facilities must be available for professional training, both initial and continuing, to ensure that an adequate standard of knowledge, expertise, and practice is attained and maintained. Formal certification of training and accreditation to practice is recommended
- *Workload:* a sufficient number of trained anaesthetists must be available so that individual doctors may practice to a high standard. Time must be allocated for professional development, administration, research, and teaching

---

repeated haphazardly and unnecessarily as the incumbent moves from hospital to hospital. Attempts to structure training have been made in some regions by the establishment of carefully constructed rotational training programmes which are closely monitored and during which the progress of the trainees is carefully assessed at regular intervals.

The Royal College of Anaesthetists plays an important part in maintaining standards by "recognising" hospitals as being suitable for training a specified number of senior house officers and registrars.[9] At present hospitals are categorised as either schedule 1 or schedule 2, the difference being that those in schedule 2 offer a more extensive range of experience. The College appoints a Visitor, who is a member of the College Council, to make the inspection. Such visits are carried out every five years, or earlier if a serious problem is detected. The College suggests to the host department that the regional postgraduate dean, local managers, and those responsible for postgraduate medical education are invited to be present for part of the visit. Hospitals seeking recognition submit applications on a prescribed form so that information about facilities, staffing, resources, and problems are available before the visit. Confidential interviews with the junior staff in addition to discussions with consultant staff are a normal part of these visits. The Visitor makes an assessment of the overall clinical experience to be gained by the trainees, the general facilities available (including anaesthetic rooms, operating theatres, recovery rooms, and intensive care areas), the adequacy and standard of staffing (including the consultant:trainee ratio), and a survey of the overall programme of education and associated facilities (such as adequacy of provision of books, journals, and library facilities).

The Visitor's report is received by the College's Hospital Recognition Committee (which has cross representation with the Recognition Committees of the Royal College of Surgeons of England and the Royal College of Obstetricians and Gynaecologists) and which makes recommendations to the Council of the Royal College of Anaesthetists. In cases that are not straightforward the Council may ask for further information, or for a follow up visit by the Regional Educational Adviser, or even another formal inspection. It must be emphasised that the decisive factor in granting recognition is evidence of the willingness and ability of consultants to educate their trainees and of adequate opportunity of study for those in the training grades. Although the object of the exercise is to identify suitable posts for basic specialist training the Visitor sometimes finds time-expired doctors occupying such posts for long periods; the implication is that these people are there to do service work with practically little or no attempt to improve their knowledge. This is where Regional Postgraduate Deans have an important part to play in ensuring that precious training posts are occupied by legitimate trainees.

Higher specialist training

The Joint Committee for the Higher Training of Anaesthetists (JCHTA) is responsible for overseeing the adequacy of training of senior registrars in much the same way as the Hospital Recognition Committee does for senior house officers and registrars. The JCHTA consists of representatives of the Royal College of Anaesthetists, the Scottish Standing Committee of that College, the Faculty of Anaesthetists of the Royal College of Surgeons in Ireland, the Association of Anaesthetists of Great Britain and Ireland, and the Association of University Professors of Anaesthesia. The scheme of training is designed to help the prospective consultant anaesthetist obtain the best possible training and to have access to the best available advice in pursuing it (box 5).[10]

Three years is the minimum time spent in higher specialist

Box 5 – Terms of reference of the JCHTA

- To keep under general review the general working of the scheme of higher anaesthetic training
- To consider and advise on matters of policy relating to the scheme
- To keep appropriate bodies informed of the progress of the scheme
- To draw up, after inspection, a list of approved posts, and to keep these under review
- To keep a roll of trainees
- To recommend to the appropriate College or Faculty that a Certificate of Accreditation be issued to those candidates who have completed an approved period of training
- To give advice to consultants or trainees on individual variations from approved programmes

---

training although some senior registrars remain in post for longer periods. The training provides experience in those aspects of anaesthesia to which the trainees did not have adequate exposure during their time in basic training. It is possible for trainees, however, once they have obtained senior registrar posts and have enrolled with the JCHTA, to apply for a maximum of one year's retrospective credit in respect of duly considered time spent in the registrar grade since obtaining the Fellowship diploma. Furthermore, the period of higher specialist training offers the prospective consultant progressively increasing responsibility and the opportunity to undertake, under consultant supervision, all the duties that will eventually be discharged independently. The content of the training encompasses not only the necessary clinical experience but also experience in teaching, management, research methods, and administration; senior registrars are encouraged to spend a block period of a year abroad or in research.

Higher specialist trainees become proficient in major specialty work, such as anaesthesia for cardiothoracic, neurological, and major paediatric surgery, as well as developing further expertise in the relief of pain, obstetric anaesthesia and analgesia, and intensive care. Nevertheless, it is not possible for a senior registrar to become completely proficient in every aspect of every subspecialty of anaesthesia during this time. The prospective consultant who aims at a particular future subspecialty interest needs to obtain further experience by a prolongation of the minimal training period, by secondment, or both. The period of higher specialist training is important for fostering the commitment of trainees towards the advancement of knowledge in the specialty, and the JCHTA regards it as vital to encourage young anaesthetists to consider an academic career and recognises that special arrangements have to be made with academic departments in this respect.

When a trainee has completed the designated period of higher specialist training the JCHTA asks for a report from the consultant in charge of training to the effect that the period of training has been completed satisfactorily, providing details of the trainee's exposure to highly specialised experience, and stating that the trainee may be regarded as satisfying the minimum requirements for the assumption of consultant status. When a satisfactory report has been obtained and assessed by the JCHTA that body recommends to the appropriate College or Faculty the granting of a Certificate of Accreditation, so accreditation represents a clear recognition by the College or Faculty that the holder is eligible for consultant appointment. Nevertheless, the statutory Advisory Appointment Committees which govern appointments to consultant posts are not obliged to appoint only those holding Certificates of Accreditation. There has been a problem for some years with respect to reconciling the periods of training in the United Kingdom with those in Europe. Hopefully this matter will soon be resolved following discussions between the European Community (EC), the General Medical Council, and the Chief Medical Officer of the Department of Health and his advisory body.[11]

Part time training

The Department of Health offers a scheme to enable certain doctors to undertake part time training. This is known as the scheme for *Doctors with domestic commitments* (PM(79)3) and it attracts mainly women doctors with families. Unfortunately there is only a limited number of posts available under the scheme, which is subject to the overall manpower requirements of the specialty. There has always been a bottleneck between the basic and the higher specialist training grades as too many registrars continue to chase too few senior registrar positions.[12] Indeed, about half the doctors qualifying from medical schools in the United Kingdom at present are women, and so the problem can be expected to be worse than 13 years ago when Edmonds-Seal *et al* reported.[13] In one respect at least conditions have improved somewhat as the Royal College of Anaesthetists no longer requires a doctor training, say, half time, to double the anticipated usual period in achieving accreditation.

Role of examinations in training

Examinations have been an integral part of specialist training in the United Kingdom for many years although they have not been used in some European countries, where completion of a satisfactory training period has been regarded as more important. The Diploma of Anaesthetics (DA) established in 1935 was complemented in 1953 by a two part examination (primary and final) for the Diploma of Fellowship of the Faculty of Anaesthetists in the Royal College of Surgeons of England (FFARCS); the standard in this examination is equivalent to that of fellowships in the other specialities. In 1985 the Fellowship was converted into a three part examination whereby a pass in the first part conferred a DA as long as the successful candidate completed a minimum of one year's training in a duly recognised hospital in the United Kingdom. The important sphere of the basic sciences (physiology and pharmacology) forms part 2 of the Fellowship examination and the final tests all aspects of anaesthetic practice. Nevertheless, a three part examination is out of step with the other specialities and indeed in my view needs to be reformed because important areas such as physics, clinical chemistry, and measurement (and to some extent anatomy) have been accorded less importance than they should have in the process.

For many years British anaesthetists holding the FFARCS (now the FRCA) diploma have been highly regarded, but the superiority of the British trained anaesthetist – if it ever existed – could have well resulted from the much longer period of training in the United Kingdom than other countries.[14] There is, however, a growing acceptance that examinations are a useful evaluative tool in anaesthetic training; several countries (Sweden, Norway, and Switzerland) which used not to have examinations have now adopted the examination (EAA diploma) of the European Academy of Anaesthesiology. The importance of examinations in the quality of care cannot be overestimated and their importance lies in the potent influence they have over training and motivation for study. A large amount of the education which is offered to postgraduates is therefore oriented specifically towards the needs of the examination. The examination should be designed to test that the objectives of training have been met and it has been argued that this is only feasible at the end of training when the full range of core objectives have been met.[15] A recent study of surgical students at the Flinders University of South Australia found that when no clear guidelines and course objectives were given in a self-directed learning programme, the student – far from exploring the topic widely and pursuing personal interests – tried to guess what would feature in the final examination and concentrated on that.[16]

Written papers may be useful tests of factual knowledge but are poor at assessing clinical skills. Assessment of clinical competence presents difficulties but the problems are not insuperable. At present, the final part of the FRCA examination includes a clinical section in which the candidates take a history and make a physical examination of volunteer patients with various medical diseases. Obviously some patients cannot be brought to the examination centre though, because of the numbers of candidates involved, there has been a shift in part towards examining some candidates in hospitals. A form of "in house" assessment in their own hospital might be better provided there were adequate safeguards. Though real patients have traditionally been used in both undergraduate and postgraduate assessment an alternative (the simulated or standardised patient) was introduced by Barrows in 1964 and this concept has been further developed.[17]

A carefully thought out objective structured clinical examination (OSCE)[18 19] may be a good way to assess essential clinical skills though there are logistical problems[20]; despite its structured format it is essential that it is indeed objective. The OSCE was introduced in the late 1970s and used by the police force for promotional assessment, and in some institutions for examining medical students. The objectives of the test are identified and recorded; the OSCE is then designed to cover all the required areas. The candidates rotate around a series of "stations", at each of which they are asked to do a clinical task or to answer questions on material provided. Assessors are present at the relevant stations to assess the candidates' performance with standard checklists. Clinical models and simulated patients can be used during OSCEs to allow large numbers of candidates to be tested on the same clinical problem without tiring or distressing real patients.

Marking can be completed as the OSCE proceeds and prompt feedback is possible. OSCEs are easy to mark with optical mark readers and allow testing of skills that traditional methods ignore. Nevertheless, the OSCE is not the answer for the assessment of complex performance; rigid examination structures are inappropriate for clinical tasks requiring eclectic, responsive skills that are controlled by clinical judgement.[21] The Royal College of Anaesthetists will introduce the OSCE in place of the traditional clinical examination in the final part of the FRCA from June 1994. The format of part 3 will continue to include a paper of multiple choice questions, a written paper, and two 30 minute oral examinations, one of which consists of structured questions, each with two examiners. It is envisaged that the new OSCE will consist of 12 "stations" at each of which the candidate spends five minutes with a 90 second gap between stations so that the whole round takes just under 80 minutes. An overview of the process has been presented by Hewitt and Hatch.[22] OSCEs alone are not particularly reliable, but combined with other components they do increase the reliability and validity of the examination structure.

The use of training simulators has been pioneered in anaesthesia by Gaba.[23] The idea is not new; indeed, quintains were objects used as surrogate enemies in Roman times for training soldiers.[24] Human error is thought to play a part in most anaesthetic accidents and exposure of trainees to simulated critical incidents is useful.[25 26] Although simulators are both interesting and expensive the main disadvantage is that competition for places on the simulators means that any one person receives limited exposure. The future of simulation of acute clinical skills which is most important in the training and assessment of anaesthetists may lie in the computer concept of "virtual reality."

The FRCA examination takes place towards the end of basic specialist training and must be passed before higher training can start. It is not an exit examination (unlike the EAA) so the higher aspects of training are not formally examined as basic specialist training is. The examination is, however, correctly placed in the overall scheme of training for it combines the elements of the two approaches – an examination of the skills completed during the basic specialist period plus an assessment (in the form of a Certificate of Higher Training) covering the senior registrar period.

Problems with present training of anaesthetists

Training is often seriously prolonged and inefficient despite the fact that under the present arrangements the training of an anaesthetist should be completed in a minimum of six years if no time is lost.[27] There are many anaesthetists still in posts from which they have obtained the maximum training experience but have not been able to secure the next post up the ladder. It should be possible to produce a well trained safe anaesthetist in five years rather than six without compromising quality or standards, given that overlap is minimised and that the doctor can progress without hindrance through the relevant training grades. This objective can be realised only by structural revision of the training grades, by adjusting present working patterns to emphasise the importance of education and training over pure service work, and the reversion from a three part to a two part FRCA diploma examination. Radical thinking and changes such as these will be required to bring the United Kingdom into harmony with the EC in terms of specialist registration; only three years' training is presently required as the minimum for full-time training in anaesthesia in the EC. The problem of the recognition in the United Kingdom of specialised qualifications obtained in other member states of the EC has brought matters to a head and will soon be resolved.

Specialist training and the European Community

The European Commission had expressed concern that the existing system in the United Kingdom for the mutual recognition of specialist medical qualifications with our European partners might not comply fully with the 1975 directives. The Commission's views were, firstly, that there would be an infringement if the United Kingdom were not to recognise other member states' certificates as being evidence of completion of specialist training, and secondly that if the United Kingdom certificate was awarded at an intermediate point during postgraduate training rather than at completion it would be contrary to the directive. Accordingly in 1992 the Secretary of State set up a working group under the chairmanship of the chief medical officer at the department of health, Dr Kenneth Calman, to advise on any action needed to bring the United Kingdom into line with the EC directives on medical training.

The working group reported in 1993 and its report is generally known as the *Calman report*.[28][29] Its main recommendations are shown in box 6. The report states that the award of a Certificate of Completion of Specialist Training (CCST), or an equivalent qualification from another member state, should be indicated in the medical register by the letters "CT" together with the relevant specialty, the year of the award, and the state in which the qualification was awarded. The *Calman report* was accepted by the government at the end of 1993, but no additional funds were allocated to implement it

Continuing medical education (CME) for senior staff

It is simply not possible for a physician, having gained a consultant appointment or its equivalent, to become buried in clinical practice and rely solely on experience if society is to be provided with a high standard of medical care for the ensuing 25–30 years.[30] Both the Government and the General Medical Council have expressed a wish to see evidence that consultants continue to educate themselves and modernise their practice throughout their working life, and new arrangements are in place to define budgets for postgraduate education and CME in the regions: the budget for postgraduate education is now held by the regional postgraduate

---

Box 6 – Main recommendations of the Calman report

- Introduction of improved training grades by the end of 1995
- Establishment of a single training grade by mid 1995 to replace career registrar and senior registrar grades. This intriduces the concept of continuous ("seamless") training: the working group nevertheless recognises the distinction between completion of specialist training and continuing medical education which should continue throughout a doctor's career
- Introduction of a new Certificate of Completion of Specialist Training (CCST) to be awarded by the General Medical Council on the advice of the relevant medical Royal College. A doctor who had been awarded a CCST would be allowed to practice independently and would be eligible for appointment as a consultant within the NHS
- The establishment of regular discussions between educational bodies and postgraduate deans as soon as possible

---

dean and those for CME at unit level.[31] Though it seems that the medical profession lags behind other professional groups in failing to keep abreast of changes in a formal and regulated way, Professor Michael Rosen, Past President of the Royal College of Anaesthetists, produced guidelines on CME for anaesthetists in 1991. These followed publication of the NHS Management Executive (NHSME) document in March 1991 in which proposals for CME for consultant and other career anaesthetists were made. There have been clear indications from the General Medical Council that it wished to see quinquennial reaccreditation. The NHSME accepts in principle that CME is valuable to the NHS, and that it should be recognised as a fair charge against contracts and required in trusts as well as in district managed units.

Most anaesthetists believe that the time is long overdue when the specialty must be able to show that it is making every effort to maintain competence. The Conference of Medical Royal Colleges and their Faculties has discussed the questions of reaccreditation and recertification, which may be voluntary, contractual, or mandatory, and may be required every three to five years. The retention of a CT entry on the Medical Register to signify that an anaesthetist has been fully trained may in future depend on CME. It will be a condition for employment, and therefore by implication the employer will accept finance responsibility for it.

The Royal College of Anaesthetists and the other Colleges have been invited to introduce a system of CME;[32] indeed this is a positive and preferred course of action because the College is better able to do this effectively than other bodies – for example, regional postgraduate deans or the General Medical Council itself.

The object of CME is to ensure that anaesthetists keep up to date with advances in the basic sciences and in the clinical practice of anaesthetics relevant to their work. CME is defined as the education of anaesthetists in permanent posts – that is, consultants – but those in staff grade and associate specialist posts will have to be considered urgently.[33] Many doctors in sub-consultant grades have a narrow experience of the specialty, are supervised little if at all, get set in their ways and are resistant to change, and do not have access to – or do not take advantage of – opportunities for postgraduate education.

Type of education
- Audit of clinical practice

41

- Lectures (particularly with strong audience participation)
- Courses
- Workshops
- Conferences
- Self-assessment exercises including distance learning by satellite television, videotapes and audiotapes, and computer assisted learning (Though self-assessment and distance learning are of great benefit to the individual they do not intrinsically lend themselves to outside appraisal)

Level of education

- Hospital or district
- Regional
- National and international
- In the home by new technology

Organisers of education

- Tutors, regional advisers, and recognised teachers of the Royal College of Anaesthetists
- Medical schools (universities) and postgraduate deans
- Associations, academies and colleges (national and international)

Assessing the quality of education

The education listed above can be acceptable only if there is some method of vetting its quality and this will have to be done at various levels. At first, it must be done centrally by the Royal College but later possibly by regional groups acting according to College Guidelines.

Quality can be monitored by:

- Reviewing the content of courses and conferences with regard to the balance among research, basic science, clinical progress, review, revision topics, and so on. The subjects and the background of the teachers usually give a broad indication of the value of a course.
- Reviewing the course material provided by lecturers and organisers – for example, lectures notes, references, abstracts, and tapes.
- Reviewing formal end of course assessments by those attending – for example, quality of lecture content, quality of lecturing, topicality, clarity, and feed back to lectures.

These means of assessing quality have been used by the College for many years for courses organised both centrally and peripherally.

Assessing the effect on the consultant

This is the most difficult factor to measure. For most local education, including audit, it may have to be assumed that the duration alone rather than the quality of exposure has some effect, but this will have to be recorded and so consultants should keep a record or log book of their educational activities. Some consultants already keep a note of such activities on their *curricula vitaes*. The Royal College of Physicians of Edinburgh has proposed the organisation and coordination of College teams of Clinical Unit Visitors to ensure that there is appropriate CME activity in local hospitals.[34] These teams would be widely representative of the College Fellowship and include relevant specialist groups as required. It is important that two cultures do not develop; those who do the visiting or inspections must be treated similarly in turn.

Lectures, courses, and conferences can be assessed from their programmes and may be allocated credit hours (or cognitive points, which is the term the Royal College of Obstetricians and Gynaecologists uses[35]), once again assuming that exposure as well as quality has an effect. This system is accepted in the United States and may be regarded as the "softest option" of the various possibilities for the United Kingdom (the "hardest option" being formal re-examination). This should be the least that is done for CME although its effectiveness is debatable (box 7).

Reaccreditation

If the above, and any other activities further considered, are thought to be suitable educational activities then the reaccreditation body will need to define the minimum standard to be attained by each method of education before granting approval. The minimum participation required for reaccreditation – for example, number of audit meetings, lectures, conferences, number of credit hours required, and, if introduced, the pass mark of the five yearly multiple choice questionnaire – will then have to be agreed. For any single person it will be essential to ensure that reduplication of CME does not occur so that the overall number of credit hours is satisfied but the breadth of necessary exposure in the specialty and related skills is not attained.

Failure

What is to be the fate of those who do not achieve the reaccreditation criteria? A further year may be granted in the hope that they can meet the necessary standard. Distance learning programmes would obviously benefit those who are geographically isolated. Access to medical libraries, or data and information acquisition terminals, or both, is essential. Failure, however, demands personal help from a colleague who can provide personal tuition and counselling. Moreover it is difficult to cope with failure unless adequate support and help from colleagues or other people is available. Failure of a unit or department to meet the required

---

Box 7 – Types of assessment of CME

- Self assessment by multiple choice questions, videotapes, and audiotapes
- Use of simulators to test the acute skills needed in the specialty
- Credit for satisfactory completion of approved courses of instruction – for example, Advanced Trauma Life Support (ATLS)
- Central assessment through log books, credit hours, and multiple choice questionnaires leading to reaccreditation every five years
- Methods of certifying participation in educational activities (by tutors, advisers, and course advisers)
- Certificates of credit hours (or cognitive points) on course completion
- Results of self assessment

---

standards of CME should ultimately result in the removal of that unit's accreditation to train junior staff. At present, removal of College or JCHTA recognition from a hospital for basic or higher specialist training. respectively, may be done (and has) through the process of the five yearly visits; nevertheless, apart from the loss of face at the institution involved, the competition for junior posts in anaesthetics has been such that doctors continue to apply for these unrecognised posts. If the consultants themselves fail to achieve sufficient CME then that institution should cease to be recognised for the training of junior staff. If an individual consultant fails to satisfy the requirements for participation in CME then ultimately his name should be removed from the specialist register of the General Medical Council; such an instance is likely to be rare.[34]

Study leave

It is important to ensure that all consultants take up their full allocation of study leave. This is at present only 30 days allowed over three years. It is regrettable that many consultants do not take their full allocation. In contrast, in the United States it is expected that anaesthesiologists complete the number of credit hours that are necessary as prescribed by the state licensure, and the employing hospitals or departments pay for it. It is arguable that those wholly in private practice have less incentive to pursue CME, but nevertheless many such practitioners belong to group private practices and so can organise the necessary free time.

Consultants from outside the United Kingdom

Consultant anaesthetists entering posts in the United Kingdom from abroad who do not possess the necessary minimum requirements of CME would either need to undergo some form of re-examination or else be given a "period of grace." Interactions with the EC regulations governing the free movement of doctors will need to be taken account of, because CME is not a general requirement at present in member states. It would be greatly advantageous if the provision of CME could be made uniform throughout the EC, and indeed throughout Europe as a whole in due course.

Administration

Any CME scheme requires a secretariat and database to record the "good standing" of consultants centrally in the form of records of credits, courses attended, and date of reaccreditation. Reaccreditation would be calculated from the date of specialist registration with the General Medical Council.

A database of all recognised courses will be necessary. External course programmes would be submitted to a panel of advisers of the College, such as its Education Committee, and such courses and lectures would then be advertised as attracting a number of credits. The panel of advisers might need to include representatives from other regional or national bodies concerned with the education of anaesthetists. It is possible that postgraduate deans may wish to become involved. After each course participants would be issued with a certificate indicating the number of credits awarded, plus a form on which confidential comment may be made to the College about the organisation and effectiveness of the course.

Conclusions

There should be harmony with the CME requirements of the other specialities. The Royal College of Anaesthetists intends to introduce a scheme as soon as possible, as will the other Royal Colleges, and this could be achieved by ensuring that the standards of reaccreditation were not pitched at too high a level in the first instance. Intense monitoring of the process will be required and constraints applied as the scheme progresses. It is essential that consultants take their minimum allocation of study leave and that this is fully funded. It might be preferable to begin the CME scheme gradually, for instance it might start with older practitioners, say initially those aged 50 and over, and progress in steps of five years to younger colleagues as the momentum develops. Alternatively, it could start with the younger consultants and work up.

The need for CME amongst non-consultants in permanent or semipermanent non-training grades is also vital and should be organised in a similar manner.

Sources of funding and the costs of the CME exercise have not been definitely worked out, but it is likely that the main source of income would be met from the reaccreditation fees. Colleges would need to be reimbursed for undertaking this. It is believed that fundholding authorities would not wish themselves to be involved in reaccreditation.

I thank Professor M Rosen and Professor M D Vickers of Cardiff for helpful discussions, the President of the Royal College of Anaesthetists for permission to quote from the College's publications *Basic Specialist Training* and *Higher Specialist Training*, and the President of the European Academy of Anaesthesiology for permission to include extracts from the Academy's publication *Objectives of Training* by Professor M D Vickers and Professor A P Adams.

1 Vickers MD. Syllabus: objectives of training. In: *Teaching and training in Europe*. London: European Academy of Anaesthesiology, 1988:25–32.
2 European Academy of Anaesthesiology. *The aims and objectives of education and training in anaesthesiology and intensive care*. London: European Academy, 1992.
3 *Objectives of training, examinations and continuing medical education*. Melbourne: Australian and New Zealand College of Anaesthetists, 1992.
4 Thames Postgraduate Deans. *A strategy for postgraduate medical and dental education in the Health Service*. London: British Postgraduate Medical Federation, 1990.
5 Statement. *Educational aspects of working in hospitals*. London: Council of the Royal College of Anaesthetists, 1990.
6 Sykes WS. *Essays on the first hundred years of anaesthesia*, Vol. 2. Edinburgh: Churchill Livingstone, 1961:26–43.
7 Norman J. Education in safety. *Br J Anaesth* 1987;**59**:922–7.

8 International standards for a safe practice of anaesthesiology. *Eur J Anaesthesiol* 1993;**10**(Suppl 7):12–15.

9 *Basic specialist training guide.* London: Royal College of Anaesthetists, 1991.

10 *Higher specialist training.* London: Joint Committee for Higher Training of Anaesthetists, 1990.

11 *Specialist medical training in the UK.* London: Department of Health, 1992. (PL/CMO(92)13).

12 The 1980 Annual Conference of Linkmen of the Association of Anaesthetists of Great Britain and Ireland. *Anaesthesia* 1981;**36**:102.

13 Edmonds-Seal J, Eaton JW, McNeilly RH. Part-time training for doctors with domestic commitments (DDC). *Anaesthesia* 1980;**35**:1027.

14 Vickers MD. The role of examinations in specialist training. In: *Teaching and training in Europe.* London: European Academy of Anaesthesiology, 1988:50–7.

15 Vickers MD. Evaluation of training: the role of examinations. In: Lunn JN, ed. *Quality of care in anaesthetic practice.* London: Royal Society of Medicine, 1984:264–77.

16 Prideaux DJ. 'We are only interested in the Exam'. Assessment and self directed learning in medical education. In: Harden RM, Hart IR, Mulholland H, eds. *Approaches to the assessment of clinical competence, Part 1.* 5th Ottawa Conference on Assessment of Clinical Competence, 1992. Dundee: University of Dundee and Centre for Medical Education, 1993:90–5.

17 Barrows HS, Abrahamson S. The programmed patient: a technique for appraising student performance in clinical neurology. *Journal of Medical Education* 1964;**39**:802–5.

18 Harden RMcG, Stevenson M, Downie WW, Wilson GM. Assessment of clinical competence using objective structured clinical examination. *BMJ* 1975;**i**:447–51.

19 Harden RM, Gleeson FA. Assessment of clinical competence using objective structured clinical examination. *Med Educ* 1979;**13**:41–54.

20 Lowry S. Assessment of students. *BMJ* 1993;**306**:51–4.

21 Cox K. No Oscar for OSCA. *Med Educ* 1990;**24**:540–5.

22 Hewitt PB, Hatch D. Objective structured clinical examination of anaesthetists. In: Harden RM, Hart IR, Mulholland H, eds. *Approaches to the assessment of clinical competence, Part 1.* 5th Ottawa Conference on Assessment of Clinical Competence, 1992. Dundee: University of Dundee and Centre for Medical Education, 1993:295–8.

23 Gaba DM. Improving anesthesiologists' performance by simulating reality. *Anesthesiology* 1992;**76**:491–4.

24 Good ML, Gravenstein JS. Anesthesia simulation and training devices. *Int Anesthesiol Clin* 1989;**27**:161–8.

25 Schwid HA, O'Donnell D. Anesthesiologists' management of simulated critical incidents. *Anesthesiology* 1992;**76**:495–501.

26 Gaba DM, deAnda A. The response of anesthesia trainees to simulated critical incidents. *Anesth Anal* 1989;**68**:444–51.

27 Healy TEJ. *Plan for assessment and structured training of anaesthetists.* Training Methods Working Party. London: Royal College of Anaesthetists, 1992.

28 Report of a working group on specialisr medical education. *Hospital doctors: training for the future.* London: HMSO, 1993.

29 Repoort to the chief medical officer's working group to advise on specialist training in the United Kingdom. *Training for specialist practice.* London: HMSO, 1993.

30 Toft AD. *Preface. Continuing medical education for trained physicians.* Edinburgh: Royal College of Physicians, 1992:1.

31 *Postgraduate and continuing medical and dental education.* London: Department of Health, 1990. (EL(90)179).

32 Report of a working party. *Continuing medical education.* London: Royal College of Anaestists, 1993.

33 Working Paper. *Educational needs of the staff grade.* London: Standing Committee on Postgraduate Medical Education (SCOPME), 1992.

34 Council Committee on Education. *Continuing medical education for trained physicians.* Edinburgh: The Royal College of Physicians of Edinburgh, 1992:13.

35 *Report of the RCOG Working Party on continuing medical education.* London: Royal College of Obstetricians and Gynaecologists, 1991.

4 Medical audit and resource management in anaesthesia

A G H COLE

There have been enormous advances in medical technology during the past 25 years and as a result the number of complex and intricate procedures that can be done successfully has mushroomed; costs have risen in a similar way.

Society's expectations of medical care have increased as fast as the advances in medical technology, both with regard to access to the most up to date technology and to equality of that access. Society also expects the highest quality of care and its previous tolerance and goodwill concerning medical mishaps has all but disappeared.

These changes demand that resources must be managed as effectively as possible, and that downward pressure on costs should not result in reduced quality.

The connection between these two is plain – if one can reduce costs and maintain quality then there is an improvement in cost-effectiveness. It is, however, necessary to measure medical practice and its quality if it is to be protected from overenthusiastic management of resources. This is the task of medical audit.

Medical audit is a relatively new term, but the concept of measuring medical practice is nearly as old as the profession itself. Case conferences, necropsies, and the discussion of results in professional journals have long been an important part of medical practice. The reasons that this process has been formalised by giving it the name "medical audit" are shown in box 1.

Medical audit is focusing attention on a part of medical practice that has traditionally been accepted but not universally applied and not previously defined. It can be defined as "The systematic and

Box 1 – Reasons for medical audit

- The quality of medical practice can be maintained and improved only if it is measured and reviewed constantly and comprehensively
- The process must be applied systematically and in a structured rather than a haphazard way
- The profession and the nation must protect the quality of its health service from the pressures of cost
- Society has demanded that there is accountability within the health care professions for quality and the management of risks

critical analysis of the quality of medical care including the procedures for diagnosis and treatment, the use of resources, and the resulting outcome and quality of life for the patient."[1]

Resource management is also a comparatively new term in health care. The name implies the establishment of cost-effectiveness and there is no doubt that this is its ultimate aim. It is, however, a term that has been coined in the NHS by an information system project that collects and collates data about patients, diagnostic and therapeutic coding, and costing. The object is to provide information to enable better decisions to be made about the application of resources – consequently it is often seen as a management tool.

The most obvious link between medical audit and resource management is their overlapping requirements for information. A master patient index is a first essential for resource management and such an index is of considerable value for providing background data for medical audit. Accurate diagnostic and therapeutic information is vital for both activities, although there are differences in the requirements for detail and timeliness.

The most important connection is the link between quality and cost. A quality product or service has to marry the provision of excellence with cost-effectiveness, because in a resource limited world cost can be measured against other benefits that may be foregone. Medical audit therefore, which is a medical form of quality assurance, must consider the audit of costs as part of its task. Taking this idea to an extreme, a real enthusiast for the benefits of the market place might go so far as to say quality (medical audit) and resource management are indivisible.

Medical audit

The purest form of audit measures the effects of medical management on outcome, but outcome is difficult to measure in medicine. There are enormous variations between patients in the natural history of disease and in healing; outcomes are often indistinct. It is therefore necessary to audit the process of medical practice to maintain quality. Process is complex and multi-faceted, which underlines the need for medical audit to be structured and systematic if it is to be comprehensive.

Processes of medical practice are not confined to the techniques of diagnosis and treatment, but include all aspects of medical care (box 2).

Box 2 – Aspects of audit of process

- Hospital facilities
- Organisation and structure of medical practice
- Medical staffing
- Other staff
- Training
- The audit process itself

Medical audit entails monitoring practice, often by peer review of the data. Such a review requires standards against which care can be measured so medical audit is often described as being cyclical (figure 1).

Collection of data

Data can be collected manually but computers have made this task potentially much easier. It is the advances in information technology that have made much of medical audit possible, but often considerable work is necessary before useful information can be retrieved. The commonest mistake is to collect too much information; this results in a massive database which is difficult to interpret. It is relatively easy to put data into a database, but time consuming to retrieve it. Enthusiasm for computer technology sometimes results in the data collection becoming the end in itself rather than a part of the cycle.

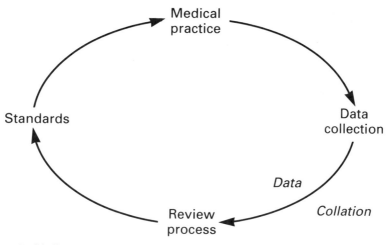

FIG 1—Medical audit cycle.

Review process

All clinicians must be a part of the review process both as subject and as a reviewer. The preparation of data for review even if the computer reports are good is time consuming, which has led to the appointment of audit assistants for the purpose.

Standards

Measurement requires standards against which to compare practice, but in medicine standards are not always easy to define. Some are set by the ethical code of society (particularly those regarding life, death, and human suffering), and others have to be agreed by the profession itself; some may be written, while others are a question of judgment unique to each case. Written standards in medicine are important but cannot be comprehensive; they also change as medical knowledge and society changes.

Size of the audit group

Because medical audit involves peer review, it follows that audit is a group activity. The larger the group the more reliable are any statistics generated but the less detailed are the results, which makes it less useful for individual interpretation. To realise its full potential medical audit must be heterogeneous, so the size of the group will vary according to the type of audit.

The Royal Colleges have taken an important role in the field of medical audit because of their statutory responsibility to maintain the quality of medical practice, and several national audits have been organised (see chapter 2). Originally district health authorities were responsible for medical audit but the development of NHS Trusts means that the responsibility will fall to them. The most natural audit groups will therefore be at specialty level in hospitals. It is, however, important to establish cross-specialty audit as well.

Types of audit

Medical audit can be compared with commercial quality assurance, in which general information is collected about a whole process and detailed analysis is confined to samples. It is the choice of these samples which is critical to the success of the programme.

General audit is the collection of data throughout the practice under scrutiny. It may include the total number of cases, and the case mix, together with the use of drugs, and treatments and operations. It is useful for giving the background and context for other audits but is generally not particularly suited to detailed review.

Morbidity and mortality audit consists of sampling those cases that had unfavourable outcomes. It is an essential audit practice, which often reveals excellent material for review and standard setting.

Critical incident audit is analagous to the aircraft "near miss" register. It is sometimes fruitful and is becoming associated with medical risk management, which makes it of increasing importance.

Key indicator audit involves the monitoring of routinely generated data to pick out cases that have varied from the norm. For example, patients with a particular diagnostic or operation code that remained in hospital longer than expected could be sampled. Unexpectedly high drug bills could also be targeted, as could patients with hospital-acquired infections, and those who were readmitted with complications. Most of these data can be generated by a resource management information system and there is obviously an area of overlap with the interests of management. Experience in the United States has suggested that it is a major source of good case material for review, and this can be of great benefit to the quality of patient care.

Topic reviews often provide the raw material for articles published in professional journals. Examples range from a study of outpatient referral patterns to the treatment in a particular disease in a certain way. There is a grey area between research and audit, but research is the discipline of improving medical care by expanding knowledge whereas audit is monitoring practice within known areas.

Random review consists of randomly sampling cases for review. It has the advantage of simplicity but because of the poor quality of medical records its usefulness can be limited. It does, however, have a considerable effect on improving medical notes and can sometimes identify major areas for quality improvement.

Patient satisfaction surveys are often difficult to interpret because of lack of objectivity but they have the advantage of measuring an outcome. They are more often part of the hospital quality assurance programme but should be considered as a medical audit activity.

Clinical freedom

A general description of medical audit cannot, however, be complete without highlighting a philosophical change that is taking place in medical practice. Doctors in the past considered clinical freedom as an absolute right to practise medicine in whatever way they saw fit within the bounds of ethical considerations. The relation between individual freedom to practise and collective responsibility is, however, difficult. Medical audit by its very nature demands that individual freedom is subject to peer review, which tends to erode that freedom. As with most dilemmas the solution must be some form of compromise. Clinical freedom to practise allows the exercise of the intellect, innovation, and flexibility which must be cherished and preserved by any professional group. On the other hand, that freedom must be controlled by the profession and subject to constant review to ensure responsible and safe delivery of care to patients.

Finally, medical audit has to be adapted to each specialty, all of which have different demands and goals. It is necessary, therefore, to examine how medical audit can be applied to anaesthesia.

Anaesthetic audit

Anaesthesia is a large specialty with a heavy case load, but the mortality and complication rate is low. This indicates that audit of outcome is likely to be both difficult and unproductive. On the other hand, the processes of anaesthesia are complex both in terms of organisation and technique so much of anaesthetic medical audit must be directed towards process. Morbidity and mortality audit is, however, the exception that proves the rule.

Morbidity and mortality audit

The confidential enquiries into perioperative deaths (CEPOD and NCEPOD) lead the way in national audit.[234] In these enquiries a proportion of all deaths within 30 days of operation were examined in detail from both surgical and anaesthetic points of view. The studies are important because they were one of the first truly national audits and crossed the boundary between specialties – inter-specialty audit is particularly relevant to anaesthesia. A forerunner of CEPOD was the triennial national enquiry into maternal mortality. This is now well established and links obstetrics and anaesthesia.[5]

Though NCEPOD produced excellent results and many useful recommendations its national viewpoint needs to be supplemented locally. Every anaesthetic department should have developed a method of identifying postoperative deaths. Officially "postoperative" deaths are those that happen within 30 days of operation, but it is sometimes difficult to record a death if the patient died after leaving hospital. Each postoperative death should be notified to the anaesthetic department and a local mechanism for review should be developed.

There are three categories of morbidity – major, intermediate, and minor.[6] Major morbidity is defined as permanent disability or disfigurement. A method for recording and reviewing all such cases should be a part of anaesthetic department policy, although it will often prove difficult to be comprehensive. It is impractical to collect all cases of intermediate and minor morbidity, and topic review is probably the most appropriate type of audit.

Critical incident survey

This technique has been used in anaesthetics.[7] The definition of a critical incident is an untoward event which may have led to harm to the patient. A system of notification of such incidents is instituted, usually on a special form which is put in a post box in theatre. Voluntary anonymity is usual.

After a few weeks of initial enthusiasm many critical incident surveys have found it difficult to maintain reliable reporting. The other difficulty is in the interpretation of the definition – it is hard to be precise. In spite of these difficulties, however, critical incident surveys have uncovered many potential dangers in anaesthesia.[8] The incidents usually fall into one or more of three categories – human error, technical failure, or patient idiosyncrasy. The capacity of critical incident reporting to show up areas of risk has attracted the attention of those involved with medical insurance and risk management. Attempts are under way to widen the scope of critical incident reporting and increase the response rate. This may lead to a conflict of interest between the profession and management if it is not handled with care.

Topic review

A well conducted audit of clinical practice in a particular field could justifiably be called research, because topic review requires the application of scientific principles. The object and methods for the review should be defined before it is started. If it is then possible to measure a definite end-point or outcome, the review becomes a clinical research project.

Local topic review can also be used to show differences in practice, stimulate discussion, and highlight any areas of peer concern. It can be a guide to future research projects and can bring attention to minor or even intermediate morbidity. Suggestions for topic reviews in a typical anaesthetic department are shown in box 3.

The list could be endless. It would be usual, however, to limit the number of topics under review at any one time so that people were not overloaded. Topic review should also cover a limited time to prevent staleness and to allow a comprehensive review of topics.

Box 3 – Suitable subjects for topic review

- Preoperative investigations
- Premedication
- Postoperative pain relief
- Use of the laryngeal mask
- Techniques of anaesthesia for a particular operation

Key indicators

Key indicators measure the incidence of certain events in an anaesthetic department and thus give a type of "health check" to the department. They can be identified either singly, in which case they are a type of critical incident reporting, or collectively. Events that might be reviewed collectively are shown in box 4.

Most of this information is usually collected from existing information systems – for example, resource management, patient administration system (PAS), the operating theatre records, and the intensive care unit records. The advantage is therefore that it does not rely on individual reporting as critical incident reporting does. The variables for reporting have to be agreed by the profession, and should be associated with departmental policies so that standards can be set and used.

Random sampling

Anaesthetic records can be chosen at random for anonymous peer review. This audit is simple, not time consuming, and has the advantage of being systematic. The main result is to point out any inadequacy of anaesthetic records, but they do improve when random samples are being taken. Preoperative assessments and American Society of Anesthesiologists (ASA) gradings improve particularly. Other results have been the discovery of some inappropriate techniques and inadequate monitoring (unpublished observations).

Box 4 – Suggested topics for key incident review

- Patients in the recovery room for more than two hours
- Unplanned transfers to the intensive care unit postoperatively
- Transfers from the day unit
- Percentage of patients who were ASA grade 4 or 5 and were anaesthetised by trainees
- Percentage of children less than 5 years old anaesthetised by consultants
- Percentage of emergencies anaesthetised by consultants
- Workload of each grade of anaesthetist
- Percentage of patients who had successful cardiac resuscitation
- Incidence of pulmonary emboli
- Cancellations of patients or lists
- High cost patients

Setting of standards

It is not possible to lay down standards for many aspects of practice, so every professional person must have their own standards and subject them to their own personal intellectual review. Many other standards are subjective so audit must be by professional discussion. Some standards, however, can be objective and agreed by a group of professionals, and to achieve consistency and quality of practice these should be written down. An anaesthetic department should collect these standards in a policy document which is available to all members of staff (box 5).

National standards may be set and a department should include these and any other standards which are suggested by other bodies, such as the guidelines published by the Association of Anaesthetists.[9]

Collection of data

Traditionally the method of collection of data in medical practice has been the contemporaneous written record. This is inadequate for medical audit because it is often inaccurate and incomplete, is usually poorly organised, and collation of pooled data would be impossibly onerous.[10] Computerisation of anaesthetic records is still being developed, but a lot of databases are too large and contain much irrelevant detail. The requirements are for pooled data which is specific and well defined.

A minimum data set has not yet been defined for anaesthesia but it is suggested that the following should be included: patient's hospital number, date of birth, and sex; ASA grade; operation code, complexity code, place, and time; name(s) and grade(s) of surgeon(s); name(s) and grade(s) of anaesthetists; and type of anaesthetic used.

Box 5 – Suggested headings for a departmental policy

- Preoperative investigation
- Grade of anaesthetist for complexity of operation
- Procedures for untoward events (for example, malignant hyperthermia and scoline apnoea)
- Level of equipment required for anaesthesia
- Level of assistance required by the anaesthetist

Most of this information is collected by the theatre management system and its database is the ideal template for the collection of data for anaesthetic audit data. Other fields may be added to support a particular topic review, and a system of flagging can be designed for critical incident review.

Collecting data for a morbidity review is more difficult to do with computers, and techniques used in research are better for this and for topic review. Hospital information systems can be helpful in collecting mortality data, though considerable investigative powers are required to establish completeness.

Review of anaesthetic audit

All members of the profession should attend audit review meetings; the attendance at such meetings can be the subject of an audit itself. It is important in anaesthesia that review is conducted not only within the department but with other specialties. One of the recommendations of NCEPOD was for interspecialty review.

Resource management

The general principle behind the recent NHS reforms was to encourage resources to follow health care activity. This is being achieved by placing hospitals in a market as a provider with external purchasers (the district health authorities and general practitioners). To continue the process, hospitals are creating internal markets, so that resources flow to departments in exchange for activity. In this context, service departments such as anaesthesia provide a service to a number of surgical "purchasers", who pay for the service from the contracts for work that they have with health care purchasers. It is essential to cost the activity of all the service departments. Unfortunately, information systems existing in hospitals in the past have been unable to support this process, which is the raison d'être of resource management.

The "case-mix" database is the electronic information system which supports resource management. It collects basic information about patients including diagnosis and treatment. To this is added information about the use of resources by individual patients which requires data from clinical departmental systems as well as the finance department.

Theatre information system

The theatre information system is one of the most important departmental feeder systems because in most general hospitals the operating theatres consume an appreciable proportion of hospital resources. Some of the essential data that need to be collected are shown in box 6.

This overlaps considerably with the information requirements of anaesthetic audit, so it is logical to use the theatre information system for the collection of anaesthetic audit data by adding the necessary extra fields. The methods for costing theatre are also similar to those used for costing the anaesthetic service.

Costing in the anaesthetic department

Costing is a two edged sword; it is an essential task if one is to control the use of resources, but it is also an expensive exercise in itself. The object, therefore, is to cost the service accurately enough to know how the money is spent without going into so much detail that it ceases to be cost effective. Attempts to cost each component of an anaesthetic and ascribe them to individual patients fall into the latter category.

It is not too difficult to establish the total cost of anaesthetic services in a hospital. There are some grey areas but as long as there is consistency it is feasible to achieve a reasonable working estimate with the finance department. The main costs are staff, drugs, consumables, and capital charges. The number of cases anaesthetised is recorded in the theatre information system, so it is then easy to calculate a crude cost/case.

This is, however, inadequate for the requirements of resource management. Some surgical departments may do operations with different ranges of complexity. The next step therefore is to refine

---

Box 6 – Essential data for theatre information system

- Patient identifier
- Surgeon
- Anaesthetist
- Operation code
- Length of time in theatre
- Use of high cost consumables

the crude apportionment with a factor which accounts for actual resources used. There are two components to this factor, the complexity and the duration of the anaesthesia. The duration is recorded in the theatre information system and a complexity value can be ascribed to each operation code. It has been suggested that a maximum of five complexity values supplemented with out of hours weighting is adequate to achieve reliable and repeatable costing. There needs to be a pilot exercise to validate how the complexity factor and duration of anaesthesia should be used to refine the cost/case apportionment.

This provides historical costing information which will support resource management and can be used as a benchmark in internal service agreements. It should be possible to produce the cost information with little delay at the end of each month, so that monitoring the agreements can be timely and accurate. There are considerable advantages in such a system for an anaesthetic department which can exercise increased control of its budget and so protect its position in the cost-conscious healthcare world.

Full autonomy can only be achieved, however, if one progresses from historical costing information to prospective pricing. Such a system would generate considerable incentives within an anaesthetic department but would demand large amounts of accurate information and a hospital would find it difficult to keep control of the prices. Most hospitals and departments will not therefore be able to evolve such a system for some years.

Medical audit and resource management (together with costing) are linked in the anaesthetic department by common data requirements. There is also the more important link that costs are an essential part of the audit process itself. The complicated triangle of costs, quality, and volume is making considerable demands on the organisation of anaesthetic departments.

Organisation of an anaesthetic department

Health care is a service business and anaesthesia is a service department within that business, and the services of the anaesthetic department have diversified and increased over the past 20 years (box 7).

In addition, the cost pressures already discussed are reflected throughout the hospital and create new challenges for the management of anaesthetic services.

Box 7 – Changes in the duties of a department of anaesthesia over the past 20 years

- Preoperative assessment has developed from a simple assessment of fitness for anaesthesia into comprehensive medical care of the surgical patient
- Relief of acute postoperative pain has diversified, developed and requires considerable expertise
- Relief of chronic pain has become a subspecialty
- Hospital intensive care has become the responsibility of the anaesthetic department
- Demands of cardiac resuscitation have grown
- There are increased responsibilities for the anaesthetist in the maternity department
- The responsibilities of the delivery of anaesthetic services to the emergency and elective surgical workload of the hospital have increased considerably during the same time
- Demands for training and education have increased in line with the demands for quality. Continuous medical education for consultants is being developed and will probably become compulsory before long

---

With such a broad area of activity it is in the best interests of anaesthetists to join together to share these responsibilities, agree local policies and share the tasks. To quote the Association of Anaesthetists "It is one of the specialty's greatest strengths – the unity of working groups of colleagues who stick by jointly agreed local policies which are in the interest of the majority."[11] To achieve this an anaesthetic department requires organisation and management on a considerable scale. In many hospitals it is appropriate to consider theatres and intensive care units within an anaesthetic directorate, and this requires a multimillion pound budget in the average sized district general hospital. This leads to the question of where the anaesthetic department should be placed in the hospital organisational structure.

The recent cost consciousness in the NHS together with the purchaser-provider split has brought considerable changes in hospital management. Firstly, there is the devolution of authority and responsibility to individual hospitals, particularly to the NHS Trusts. To gain control of finances within the hospitals, it has become essential to devolve authority and responsibility to those who commit the resources – the clinicians. This has led to the setting up of clinical directorates, which may have considerable autonomy though there has to be corporate responsibility to the hospital and the NHS.

These new management structures are evolving and the place of the anaesthetic department varies from hospital to hospital. Figure 2 shows four simple models. Model 1 shows the anaesthetic department as it has always been. Resources are given to the service by management without reference to the workload. Model 2 shows the anaesthetic department responsible for the budget for anaesthetic personnel only, with theatres and the intensive care unit within other directorates. Model 3 shows the anaesthetic department within a surgical directorate, and model 4 shows a separate directorate of anaesthesia, with theatres and the intensive care unit headed by a clinical director who is an anaesthetist. This

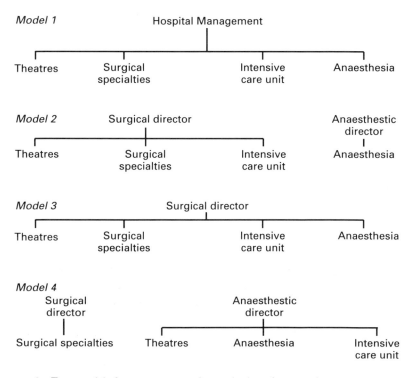

FIG 2—Four models for management of anaesthesia and surgery in an acute hospital.

clinical director has the final responsibility for providing a cost-effective service, training, audit, and negotiating a budget for the directorate according to service needs. The Association of Anaesthetists strongly favours this model which it thinks can bring substantial improvements to both hospital management and patient care.[11]

Organisation of medical audit in an anaesthetic department

Any clinical department has three main tasks: to provide a service, to undertake training and education, and to do research.

Medical audit is now the fourth task, and it includes responsibilities for reviewing standards in all activities in a department, so it is essential that it is not seen as an optional extra, but as a vital part of the fabric of a department. Final responsibility for medical audit must rest with the head of department, though it is usual to delegate it to an audit consultant who in anaesthesia should coordinate all audit activities in the department with the help of an executive committee. The size of this group and its composition depends on the size of the department – it has to decide the departmental audit structure, the areas to be audited, and the agenda for departmental audit meetings. In a large department there may be a need for an audit assistant to collect and collate the data.

Departmental audit meetings must involve all members, and other meetings should be organised with other specialties because of the team nature of our work. The frequency of the meetings should be decided locally but one audit meeting a month is a minimum. To minimise the effect on service work, some hospitals have organised rolling audit sessions that fall on different days of the week, during which all operating lists are cancelled.

The amount of time that a clinician should devote to audit is open to debate. Most consultant contracts now mention audit but it is usually less than a whole session. If one compares anaesthesia with other activities that are audited, it would seem reasonable to put aside 10% of the resources available to anaesthesia to be used for audit (box 8).

The purpose of an anaesthetist is to provide a safe and quality service to patients having operations. In modern practice, the responsibility for the delivery of that provision rests with not only the individual practitioner but also with the anaesthetic department. This collective responsibility for a safe quality service is

---

Box 8 – Amount of time that should be devoted to audit

- 5% of time of every anaesthetist (half a session/week)
- 2·5% of departmental service time for meetings
- 2·5% of departmental resources for the organisation of audit (for example, audit consultant and audit assistant)

---

delivered through the process of medical audit. In the pursuit of quality this process requires the examination of cost and volume as well as excellence. Resource management and medical audit, therefore, are closely associated.

1 Shaw CD. *Specialty medical audit*. London: King's Fund, 1992.
2 Buck N, Devlin HB, Lunn JN. *Report of a confidential enquiry into perioperative deaths*. London: Nuffield Provincial Hospitals Trust/King's Fund, 1987.
3 Campling AE, Devlin HB, Hoile RW, Lunn JN. *National confidential enquiry into perioperative deaths 1990*. London: NCEPOD (Royal College of Surgeons of England), 1992.
4 Campling AE, Devlin HB, Hoile RW, Lunn JN. *Report of national confidential enquiry into perioperative deaths 1991/1992*. London:NCEPOD (Royal College of Surgeons of England), 1993.
5 United Kingdom Departments of Health. *Report on confidential enquiries into maternal deaths in the United Kingdom 1985-7*. London: HMSO, 1991.
6 Lunn JN. Morbidity and mortality studies. In: Nimmo WS, Smith G, eds. *Anaesthesia*. Oxford: Blackwell, 1989:422–9.
7 Craig J, Wilson ME. A survey of anaesthetic misadventures. *Anaesthesia* 1981;**36**:933–6.
8 Kumar V, Barcellos WA, Mehta MP, Carter JG. An analysis of critical incidents in a teaching department for quality assurance: a survey of mishaps during anaesthesia. *Anaesthesia* 1988;**43**:879–83.
9 Royal College of Anaesthetists. *Audit in anaesthesia and the quality of practice committee*. London: Royal College of Anaesthetists, 1991.
10 Seed RF, Welsh EA. Anaesthetic records in Great Britain and Ireland. *Anaesthesia* 1976;**31**:1199–201.
11 *NHS management changes – implications for anaesthetists*. London: Association of Anaesthetists, 1992.

5 Quality in medical audit

NANCY DIXON

Medical audit – the vision and the reality

An established tradition of the medical profession is continuous self evaluation and peer review of the quality of care provided to patients, and for the past 20 years doctors have used the term medical audit to describe the process. In the United Kingdom some medical specialties have extended the principles followed in locally-based medical audits to national reviews such as the *Confidential enquiry into maternal deaths* and the *Confidential enquiry into perioperative deaths*. When the Department of Health included medical audit among the reforms of the NHS, the idea was that all doctors would take part in medical audit. The key principles included[1]:

- Medical audit involves systematic and critical analysis of the quality of medical care.
- Procedures for diagnosis and treatment, the use of resources, and the outcomes of treatment are suitable subjects for audit. The appropriateness of interventions is to be audited as well as the outcomes of such interventions.
- Peer review is fundamental. It is the mechanism by which acceptable standards of medical care will be ensured.
- The setting of acceptable standards requires specialised knowledge of current medical practice, but it is recognised that some medical interventions lack accepted measures of their efficacy.
- Medical audit functions locally, and is supported nationally by Colleges and Associations.
- Management remains responsible for ensuring that resources are used in the most effective way.

These principles include a number of assumptions about how medicine is practised and how doctors work, one of which is that most or all hospital doctors accept that all their clinical decisions can be audited; that their local colleagues will judge the quality of their work; and that the judgement of their immediate peers is what decides the quality of medical care. Other assumptions are that most doctors have acceptable standards of practice already; that clinical responsibility for the use of resources can be separated from managerial responsibility for ensuring that those resources are used most effectively; and that medical audit will result in improvements in the quality of care. The reality of the imposition of medical audit on the NHS is, however, in sharp contrast to the vision; these assumptions may not yet be valid.

Not all hospital doctors are used to cooperating with their colleagues; for many doctors, the tradition is of independence of consultants or of firms. Some doctors may need to get used to making clinical decisions as a group, and assessing whether they are consistent in their services to patients, and whether there are better ways to treat patients. Some may have to learn to consider the views of patients, families, or other practitioners about their services. In some places there may be additional social and emotional barriers to examining quality of care among peers as a result of differences in age or training, pressure of work, and in a few cases, fear of exposure.

Variations in standards and outcomes of medical practice have been analysed.[2] Some variations can be attributed to variations among the patients – for example, the severity of illness as measured by the number and complexity of coexisting conditions or the number of body systems that are physiologically affected and the extent of those effects. How much variation, however, is not known. Many observational studies of outcomes have not simultaneously examined the processes followed. A few which have done so have suggested that there may be a relationship between resources and processes and the outcome of care.[3] We cannot assume, therefore, that standards of practice are consistent among practitioners, or that standards aimed at achieving the best outcomes for the least resources are well known throughout clinical practice.

There is also some confusion about who is responsible for resources. Whether the money to run a clinical service is entrusted to a general manager or to a medical director of a clinical service is irrelevant; clinical resources are still mainly used as a result of decisions made by individual doctors. Unless doctors agree among themselves on the appropriate use of such resources and audit these agreements, neither medical nor health service management can be responsible for ensuring the most effective use of resources.

Resources are often wasted by the systems through which healthcare services are organised and operated – for example, the need to repeat an investigation because the results of the first investigation have been lost. Doctors either separately or together often feel helpless against "the system."

The final assumption (that properly conducted medical audit will result in demonstrable improvements in the quality of medical care) depends on the nature of the changes needed to achieve the improvement, the ability to achieve and maintain changes, and the control of those involved over what needs to be changed. If those who need to change are willing, and their willingness is supported by practical assistance where required, and if the change needed is under the control of those involved, medical audit can effectively improve quality. If there is no motivation to change, if the support of others is required, or if the ability to control or influence change is missing, then medical audit may not improve quality.

In summary, medical audit is a potentially powerful tool for facilitating improvements in the quality of medical care, but implementation may be limited unless there is a simultaneous commitment to additional programmes and other techniques to manage and improve quality within the entire organisation.

Medical audit as a form of quality assurance

Several definitions of medical audit have been published,[4-8] but the definitions seem to include the same components (box 1).

Several techniques for auditing have been published, and most involve one of two approaches. The first is to collect data in the absence of explicit standards to learn what present standards are, and then decide what standards should be in the light of these results. The other approach is to reach agreement on explicit standards, and then to collect data to find out the degree to which practice is consistent with these standards.[9]

Whichever approach is used, however, medical audit is ultimately quality assurance. Quality assurance is a formal continuous programme by which the quality of patient care is objectively and

---

Box 1 – Components of medical audit

- Aims to improve the quality of medical care
- Compares actual medical practice with agreed standards of practice
- Is formal and systematic
- Involves peer review
- Requires identification of variations between practice and standards; analysis of causes of such variations
- Provides feedback to those whose practices are audited
- Includes following up or repeating an audit some time later to find out if practice is fulfilling agreed standards

---

systematically measured and evaluated, and compared with an agreed standard, and problems that interfere with meeting these standards are identified and corrected. The only feature that distinguishes medical audit from any other aspect of quality assurance is peer review. Other methods of quality assurance may, but need not, incorporate peer review.

Anaesthetics in a quality assurance model

An example of audit in anaesthetics could be an audit of preanaesthetic assessment (box 2).

In a typical audit, the anaesthetists would reach agreement on what they wanted to know about their practices and would select the objectives accordingly. They would then agree on the number of cases to be included, the time period to be covered, and whether data should be collected on past, present, or future cases.

When they had agreed on the overall design, the anaesthetists would establish the standards to be used as a basis for collecting the data. One of several models for expressing standards of medical care could be followed. In the "indicator-based" approach, for example, the anaesthetists could express their objectives as shown in table I.[9]

Required elements or aspects of the preanaesthetic history are listed in the left hand column. Opposite each item, a percentage is stated of cases for which the item should be noted. In this example, all the items listed should be noted for all the patients, so the column has been omitted. Exceptions are allowable, for clinically

---

Box 2 – Objectives of an audit of preanaesthetic assessment

1 Find out whether the key aspects of the preanaesthetic history are being documented for all patients (or for a selected group of patients)
2 Ensure that findings of preanaesthetic assessments are being documented consistently by all anaesthetists
3 Confirm that preanaesthetic assessments are being carried out at the correct time
4 Find out whether results of essential investigations are available in time for the preanaesthetic assessments to be completed
5 Find out how many unnecessary investigations are being requested by anaesthetists, and what they are
6 Identify cases of disagreement among anaesthetists about patients' fitness for operation based on the anaesthetic assessment
7 Ensure that all patients have given consent for the anaesthetic to be given

---

acceptable reasons or circumstances which would justify the failure to meet the expectation stated in the percentage. A final column may be added stating the source of the data for the information required, and commonly accepted forms of notes or abbreviations, or both.

In this type of audit, the sample of cases is compared with indicators. Percentages of cases that did or did not meet the indicators are calculated. The results of the audit include these percentages, together with explanations of cases that did not meet the indicators.

The peer group of anaesthetists review the results and decide if they represent acceptable practice. They may elect to review all cases or a sample of cases that did not meet one or more indicators. Decisions would then be made by the group about whether their quality of care as represented by the audit is acceptable. If the decision is made that the standard of quality is not fully acceptable, the group must agree on improvements to be made and actions to be taken. Finally, they decide who will assume responsibility to implement the actions agreed.

Other audit objectives may require different indicators and result in different findings. For example, a wish to find out about investigations could have led to the indicators given in table II.

TABLE I   Example of medical audit of preanaesthetic assessment. The objective is to find out how well preanaesthetic assessments are being done. All aspects should be covered, with the exception of patients who are uncooperative, unconscious, or who had no records.

Aspect of care to be noted[10]	Definitions and instructions for retrieval of data
1 Note in previous and current history of presence or absence of the following: Heart or breathing problems Shortness of breath Chest pain High blood pressure Previous heart attack or rheumatic fever Fainting Epilepsy Jaundice or liver problems	See anaesthetic history for reference to all the items listed; NAD means absence
2 Previous anaesthetic history noted for: Patient Relations	
3 Family history of presence or the absence of the following serious or inherited conditions noted: Malignant hyperthermia Cholinesterase abnormalities Porphyria Dystrophica myotonica Sickle cell disease Thalassaemia	
4 Presence of false, loose, or capped teeth noted	
5 Smoking history: Smoker, yes or no If yes, how many cigarettes per day	
6 Alcohol use: Drinks alcohol: yes or no If yes, how many units per day or week	
7 Allergies noted: Allergies: yes or no If yes, name of allergens	

The examples illustrate the principles of medical audit (or quality assurance). They involve systematic and critical analysis of aspects of care provided by anaesthetists. They are concerned with procedures involved in anaesthetic care and with the use of resources. They involve a peer review process. They involve the setting of standards of practice which are acceptable to those involved, and they show how medical audit can be undertaken locally, with reference to published guidelines of practice.

The examples also illustrate what can be difficult about medical

TABLE II   Example of medical audit on preoperative investigations. The objectives are to identify unnecessary preoperative investigations and to find out if essential ones are available when required.

Aspect of care[10]	Exceptions[10]	Definitions and instructions for data retrieval
Haemoglobin concentration	None	See notes for laboratory requests
Additional laboratory investigations requested by anaesthetist	(A) Urea and electrolyte concentrations for patients over 40 years old (B) Electrocardiogram for men over 40 and all patients over 60 years old (C) Glucose concentration and chest radiograph for patients over 60 years old (D) As indicated by history	For exception D, see notes for explanation of need for investigation
Report of results of laboratory investigation available in patient's notes or sent to anaesthetist at or before time of transfer to operating theatre	Patient requires emergency operation	See notes at time patient arrives in operating theatre for results of investigations requested. An emergency operation is one done within four hours of the patient being seen by the anaesthetist

audit. The preanaesthetic assessment is one of the most common tasks that anaesthetists carry out. It can be time consuming. For most healthy patients, the risk of adverse experience that can be attributed to a failure of preanaesthetic assessment is slim. Anaesthetists accept the desirability of documenting a complete history as part of the preanaesthetic assessment, and most accept the desirability of a complete assessment of all patients, including review of the results of investigations.

Reality, however, does not always match up to what is desired. Many anaesthetists are quick to admit, even before undertaking an audit of preanaesthetic assessment, that they do not always document complete histories, that they do not request additional investigations solely in accordance with the individual patient's history, that they do not always see or know about the results of investigations before the patient is transferred to the operating theatre, and that they do not always assess all patients consistently, particularly when other pressures such as time, or the convenience of the surgeon or the patient, are involved.

The possible failure of anaesthetists to meet their own standards may not indicate either a poor attitude or lack of knowledge. An anaesthetist has various jobs to do from day to day concerning different patients in different locations. Anaesthetists may receive short notice of a task, and are occasionally requested to be in two places at once. In such circumstances anaesthetists may not feel in enough control of their time to ensure that they meet standards for all the patients all the time, particularly when they are doing a highly repetitive task which has a low risk of harming generally healthy patients.

The example of an audit assumes that there is complete agreement on the aspects of history-taking in the preanaesthetic assessment. These aspects are usually based on consensus views, but research-based evidence may not be available to support the inclusion of all the items listed in a preanaesthetic history for all patients. There is therefore an element of frustration about this approach to evaluating quality of anaesthetic care in that such an audit is aimed at achieving consistency without having a research base to indicate what is best practice.

Problems with quality assurance

Quality assurance activities, including medical audit, can

Box 3 – What quality assurance can do

- Establish a culture in which quality of service is questioned
- Provide a mechanism through which standards of practice can be discussed and agreed among the people providing the service
- Inform a service of its exact level of performance in relation to its own standards
- Identify areas of performance in which the service can be improved and suggest actions needed to improve it
- Show whether the service has been improved by undertaking follow up studies

---

achieve much for any healthcare organisation (box 3). They do, however, have some important drawbacks as a way of introducing improvements. Critics have described the approach as following the "Theory of Bad Apples," so called because the activities are aimed at searching out performance that does not comply with predetermined standards.[11]

As a model for quality improvement, quality assurance has several shortcomings.[11-15] Firstly, it relies on "quality by inspection" or "quality by checking" – that is, quality judged by direct observation or inspection of the service being provided. In medical audit, quality is usually checked by observation of entries in medical records or other documents which serve as proxy measures for direct observation of what practitioners do. This approach has been compared to that of an inspector at the end of an assembly line who decides whether goods coming off the line are to be accepted or rejected.[11]

It also tends to engender anxiety among participants as to whether they pass or fail, and practitioners may be tempted to adopt minimum or loosely-stated standards which no one is likely to fail. The experience may lead to defensive behaviour and tend to quell the search for improvement. It is not clear if professional self-evaluation and self-regulation can be effective ways of improving performance, particularly for those practitioners who have been shown to be incompetent.[15]

It assumes that standards used to check practice are the best possible standards – that is, that they will lead to the best possible results that can be achieved with the resources available. Locally-controlled medical audit programmes, however, may use different standards, but it is not clear whether each locally-determined set of standards represents care aimed at achieving the best possible outcome at the least cost.

A further implication of the model is that the causative links between processes and outcomes of medical care are known and that standards can be drawn up based on certainties about those links. Donabedian, who has written extensively about the assessment of structure, process, and outcome of healthcare, stated that "Changes in health status . . . do not serve as a measure of the quality of care until other causes for such changes have been eliminated, and one is reasonably sure that previous care is responsible for the change, which then can be truly called an 'outcome'" and also that "elements of the process of care do not signify quality until their relationship to desirable changes in health·status has been established."[16][17]

A more sensible approach to improving quality in medical care would be to recognise what is unknown about medical practice and encourage a search for scientific evidence to substantiate standards. The need to associate the assessment of medical technology with the assessment of medical quality has been recognised by the creation of a distinct form of research called "healthcare technology assessment".[18]

Measurement of quality assurance model in medical care relies heavily on documentation of information about key processes and outcomes, even though the information may be unreliable. Lack of availability of medical records is a common problem in medical audit, and computer-based clinical information systems tend to capture only views of short term clinical outcomes. Longer term outcomes or other outcomes such as behaviour modification or maintenance of a normal life style are seldom documented systematically and so are not readily retrievable for use in medical audit.

Quality assurance tends to set up a "closed loop" approach to implementing change. If audit shows that actual practice falls short of expected performance the tendency is to concentrate on raising the compliance next time. The audit becomes focused on the need to do better in the future. A review of audit findings could be used to question the systems through which people work – for example, to identify what prevents them from improving and to learn how ineffective systems could be changed. Such a use of audit, however, may require breaking out of the organisational framework of the clinical specialty in which the audit is being undertaken.

Move to quality management or continuous quality improvement

Experience with quality assurance is leading many healthcare organisations to search for alternative ways to improve the quality of their services. Principles of quality management or continuous quality improvement that differ appreciably from those of quality assurance are being introduced. These include:

- There are several ideas about what quality is, but the prevailing one should be that quality is about meeting the needs of the customer not the supplier.
- Measurement or surveillance, or both, of key processes and their

outcomes by established statistical methods can assist in the analysis of processes and systems and lead to their improvement.

- The achievement of quality depends on the interaction of many processes which are carried out by different individuals or groups who may not relate to one another in traditional terms. Understanding and control of the processes rather than the people is what is critical in quality management.

- The organisation as a whole is committed to changing processes and systems to achieve improvements in quality.

The key ideas in quality management are aimed at overcoming traditional barriers to quality assurance such as defining quality, measuring it with accepted techniques and reliable data and getting people and organisations to change their behaviour in response to these data.[19]

The American experts in quality management who influenced Japanese industrialists had a different way of expressing these ideas. Deming, for example, emphasised the need to plan a service from the customer's perspective, then carry it out according to that design, then check (audit) if it was working according to plan, and finally, to remedy any problems that were identified through auditing.[20] Juran and Gryna approached quality design by defining the quality of a service in relation to the customer's requirements for the service.[21] These perspectives both start with designing a quality service rather than auditing an existing (possibly poorly designed) system.

When Deming's "plan-do-check-act" cycle is applied to health-care organisations it shows that quality in healthcare services is seldom "designed", let alone designed from a customer's perspec-tive. Most healthcare services have evolved from systems adopted long ago in circumstances that no longer apply or from services provided in accordance with the dictates of providers. The starting point for quality management is therefore to raise basic questions about quality in relation to provision of services before measuring or analysing present levels of quality.

Continuous quality improvement ideas and tools

The principles of quality management or continuous quality improvement are supported by specific techniques, most of which can be applied in healthcare settings once a definition of quality has been agreed.[22]

Defining quality

In industry and business quality has a precise meaning: it is the totality of features and characteristics of a product or service that bear on its ability to satisfy stated or implied needs.[23] All the customer's requirements are defined explicitly for or by the supplier. Ensuring quality therefore involves all parts of an operation including design, procurement, process control, administration, finance, sales, marketing, and (where applicable) manufacture. Installation, commissioning, and decommissioning are integrated and controlled so that none is subservient to any other in the aim to meet the customer's requirements.

In business or industry it is the top manager of an organisation who accepts ultimate responsibility for directing the parts of the organisation to achieve the required quality of services or products. Maintaining quality is therefore a management function that cannot be delegated. Quality is not "bolted on" to an individual service or manufacturing process; it is a philosophy of total integration and control to achieve the required result.[24]

There is no universally accepted definition of quality as it applies to healthcare services. It must first be acknowledged that identification of the customers' requirements in healthcare is considerably more difficult than in industry.[24] True customers of healthcare services are purchasers whose views of quality are tempered by financial constraints. They usually have insufficient clinical knowledge to define their requirements, particularly those that apply to the eventual clinical and other outcomes of healthcare services. A sensitive definition of quality in healthcare may have to take into account the perspectives of the various participants in the healthcare system.[9] Providers are the most knowledgeable about technical definitions of quality, purchasers take a population-based view of quality that may involve decisions about cost-benefit or value for money decisions, and patients can express their view of the appropriateness of response to their needs including such aspects of service as communication and education.

Two definitions of quality developed for use in the United States attempted to take account of the various perspectives about quality. The US National Academy of Science Institute of Medicine developed a consensus definition as part of a national study of quality assurance programmes in American healthcare organisations: "Quality of care is the degree to which health services for individuals and populations increase the likelihood of desired health outcomes and are consistent with current professional knowledge."[25]

After the Institute of Medicine published its definition, the Joint Commission on Accreditation of Healthcare Organisations published its own definition of quality which was a modification of the Institute of Medicine definition. "Quality of patient care is the degree to which patient care services increase the probability of desired patient outcomes and reduces the probability of undesired outcomes, given the current state of knowledge." The Joint Commission's definition reflects the view that quality involves at least doing no harm to patients.[26]

One definition of quality published in the United Kingdom by the Standing Medical Advisory Committee to the Department of Health reflects the "totality of features" concept of quality. "Quality of care is an all-embracing term which encompasses everything from the patient's care to the receptionist, through the comfort of the waiting room, the effectiveness of appointment systems, the response to complaints, the nutritional quality of hospital food to clinical outcome."[27]

Patients' views of quality are now being sought in various ways, including patient surveys by written questionnaires or individual interviews. Another useful technique for use with providers, purchasers, and patients is the focus group interview.

Measuring quality by statistical techniques

Another name for measurement techniques used in quality management or quality improvement is statistical process control (box 4). The key idea is to reduce the specific or controllable variation in a process in order to improve quality.

Box 4 – Principles of statistical process control

- All work can be either counted or measured
- All work processes, when measured, have a pattern
- The pattern of work processes is likely to reveal variation
  In quality management or quality improvement, variation is identified and categorised as:
- Random – that is, not capable of attribution to any known factor – or
- Specific – that is, capable of attribution to one or more known factors

---

Descriptive and analytical statistical techniques are used to identify and attribute variation. In processes or outcomes of care, specific variations are often attributed to such factors as the severity of the patient's illness (patient-related), the years of training of the doctor involved (doctor-related), or the day or time that the patient presents for treatment (system-related).

One particular quality measurement technique is the *Pareto diagram*, which is a histogram in which data are organised by the "most-to-least" principle. The technique is based on the observation by Pareto (a 19th century economist) that 20% of the people have 80% of the wealth. The Pareto principle looks for 80% of the effect which is attributable to 20% of the causes and has become known as the 80-20 rule.

Trend charts, run charts, and *control charts* are also used to illustrate aspects of quality over time. In a trend chart, a noticeable pattern of dips or swings in mean performance over time suggests the need for further investigation. Run charts are similar to trend charts but track individual events in relation to the median of all the data in the run. Control charts are run charts that show statistically determined upper and lower limits drawn on both sides of the line illustrating mean performance. The upper and lower limits identify whether or not variations in performance are within normal limits or are "out of control."

Analysing processes

A number of techniques of quality management or quality improvement are aimed at analysing the processes involved in providing a service so that the desired requirements of the service can be met more effectively. Some of the techniques are designed to investigate processes and others are intended to use people's ideas to identify and solve problems related to quality.

A technique known as *benchmarking* is designed to help an organisation raise its standards of performance to those of the best organisation providing the same or related service. The measurable differences between ordinary performance and excellent performance are identified, then organisations which are performing at the best or excellent level are identified and their processes are analysed carefully to identify the gap between the processes that are followed in the best and in the ordinary organisations. The processes followed in the best organisation are adopted as far as possible and adapted for use by the ordinary performer to improve its own quality.

Critical incident reporting analyses particular events or incidents for the purpose of identifying how steps in the process leading up to the event can be modified to improve outcome.

Flow charts are used to draw a picture of a particular process to illustrate in sequence every activity or step in the process, with key decision-making points or options identified. In this way all those individuals involved in the overall process describe how the process works now and identify ways of improving the process.

Cause and effect diagrams are used to identify the potential causes of a problem. An example is the *fish bone* or Ishakawa analysis in which a skeleton of a fish is drawn with the head of the fish representing the effect or problem and the spines of the fish representing the potential causes. In healthcare these are usually divided into four categories: providers, patients, procedures or systems, and resources or equipment. Secondary causes can be attached to the key spines and any tertiary causes can be shown next to the pertinent secondary spines.

Making a commitment to improve quality

Nominal group process, the Delphi technique, brainstorming, affinity charts, and force-field analysis are among techniques of quality improvement that are aimed at getting those who provide services to improve the quality of the service.

The *nominal group technique* is a formal procedure for eliciting the opinions of all the people in a group to achieve consensus about problems faced by the group or actions to be taken by the group. The technique is particularly useful when attitudes may be disparate or unpopular decisions must be taken. Each member of the group lists ideas about an issue. If the group wishes to keep its answers anonymous the members list their ideas on an index card which is handed in to a facilitator. If the approach is open, each group member states the most important idea on their list and the facilitator records the idea, and the process continues until all ideas are noted. The group facilitator collects the members' responses and assists the group in setting priorities among the ideas.

The *Delphi technique* is also a formal way of obtaining opinions to achieve consensus, usually about priorities. Individual opinions are collected on questionnaires. Responses to each round of questionnaires are analysed and returned to those who replied to the questionnaires so that people can consider their ideas in relation to those of the group as a whole, and rank them. The process of circulating questionnaires or rating scales continues until clear consensus is reached.

"Brainstorming" is the collection of the maximum number of ideas on a defined subject from a group without consideration of the validity or practicality of ideas. After all the ideas have been aired they are placed in the order of priority established by the group and considered one by one. In *affinity charting*, ideas are organised into clusters of related ideas and the clusters are named.

Force-field analysis is used to help a group identify and plan how to handle forces that might influence a particular quality improvement. Driving forces are identified which are likely to favour improved performance, and restraining forces which may impede improved performance. When such forces have been identified a group can develop specific strategies to strengthen driving forces and minimise restraining forces.

The intended results of the various techniques are shown in box 5.

Quality management or quality improvement in anaesthetics

A group of anaesthetists might first consider how they and the customers and users of their services will define quality of anaes-

---

Box 5 – Results of quality management techniques

- Development of professionally and publicly acceptable definitions of quality
- Use of scientifically accepted statistical techniques to measure quality, using agreed definitions
- Thoughtful inquiry by teams of people working together about the relation between desired outcomes and routine processes used to provide them
- Emphasis on designing or redesigning healthcare services rather than continuing to accept working under ineffective systems
- Increased collaboration among professionals, patients, managers, and purchasers
- Shift in the organisation away from tradition towards a focus on quality
- Demonstrable improvements in the quality of services provided

---

thetic services. Such an analysis would consider a variety of features of quality as well as a variety of potential customers and users. Based on this analysis they would then measure their present levels of performance against the quality features listed or meet with one or more of their groups of users to discuss possible improvements in the quality of their services (table III).

A number of formal studies have measured outcomes of anaesthetic services and have reported major and minor complications.[28-31] Anaesthetists could use trend, run, or control charts to monitor the incidence of their major and minor complications, or they could "benchmark" their performance against the best reported outcomes. Alternatively, they could monitor their performance on other potential quality features such as timeliness of response to requests for epidural anaesthetics. The trend, run, or control charts would show patterns among the actual levels of quality provided by the service (fig 1). A Pareto chart could also be used to identify potential patterns; such a chart may help anaesthetists to identify the most influential problems or causes of problems or to decide which problems are worth pursuing (fig 2).

Quality management analytical techniques could be used to identify how the quality of an anaesthetic service could be

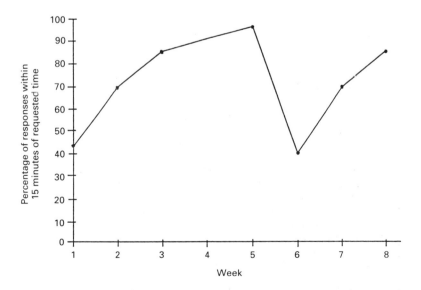

FIG 1—Response times for requests for epidural anaesthesia.

TABLE III   Possible meanings of quality in anaesthetics depending on who was asked. All groups regard safety as paramount.

Quality feature	Anaesthetists	Patients	Surgeons	Obstetricians	Psychiatrists	Other medical specialists	Nurses
Access to most experienced anaesthetists	No	No	For major trauma	For emergencies	For electroconvulsive therapy	No	For cardiopulmonary resuscitation
Appropriate anaesthetic agents used	Yes	No	No	No	No	No	No
Continuity of care by anaesthetists	No	No	No	No	No	No	For preoperative and postoperative care
Efficacy of service	Best possible outcomes	"Wake up normal"; pain control	Muscle relaxation appropriate to the procedure	No	No	No	Few minor complications requiring extra nursing care; good pain control
Timely services	No	No extra waiting	Yes	For epidural anaesthesia and caesarean sections	No	Yes	No

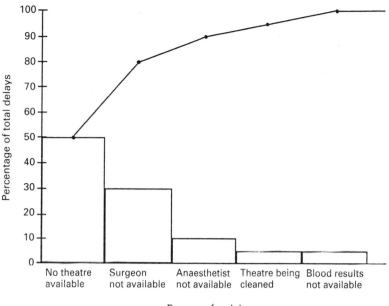

FIG 2—Chart according to Pareto's law of reasons for delay in start of emergency operations during the last three months for patients who were deemed to be fit for operation.

improved – for example, a fishbone analysis could be carried out on the findings of incomplete preanaesthetic assessments. Such an analysis could help a group of anaesthetists to identify a cluster of potential causes for which they could attempt to introduce changes (fig 3).

Flow charting of key processes could help to identify where a process or system is likely to break down under pressure, or how a system might be streamlined or simplified without compromising the quality of patient care. For example, flowcharting the process through which anaesthetists are contacted to assess or manage patients could be used to identify potential improvements in communications.

Finally, a group of anaesthetists could use consensus building techniques to agree on key elements of the service or on ways to improve the quality of the service. For example, a force-field analysis could be used to plan the implementation of a preadmission anaesthetic clinic (table IV).

TABLE IV   Implementation plan resulting from force-field analysis on preadmission clinic.

Driving forces:	Ways to strengthen:
• Safer anaesthetic care • Avoid delays attributable to waiting for results of investigations • Avoid cancellations or discharges because the patient is not fit for operation • Greater turn-around time allowed for laboratory and radiology services • Less stress on anaesthetists	• Presentation within department of data on delays, cancellations, extended stays in hospital, unanticipated discharges before operation, and possibly minor complications attributable to late or incomplete preanaesthetic assessment • Analysis of advantages to patients, anaesthetists, and managers
Restraining forces:	Ways to minimise:
• No clinic space/time available • No anaesthetist available for clinic • Concern about sudden change in patient clinical condition after clinic visit • Perceived inconvenience to patient	• Interview a small group of suitable patients • Develop protocol to identify changes in patients' condition since clinic visit • Arrange for space and an anaesthetist for a short-time trial and measure differences in delays, cancellations, patient stays, unanticipated preoperative discharges, and anaesthetists' time

From audit to continuous quality improvement

The need for and value of medical audit will continue for years to come. There is no other medical professional activity which offers the opportunity for systematic and critical discussion about standards of practice and the comparison of patterns of actual practice with such standards. A list of potential topics for audit in any medical specialty is extensive. There will be a need to follow up or repeat particular audits to confirm that practice has improved and to review and possibly revise standards as new research findings or professional guidelines appear, so the agenda for medical audit will be progressive.

Within a single medical specialty such as anaesthetics, medical audit can be usefully supplemented by quality management or improvement principles and techniques. Thinking about what quality in an anaesthetic service could mean may itself bring about some insights about how patients, colleagues, and purchasers could see the quality of service provided by the specialty. Application of accepted statistical methods to the quality of anaesthetic

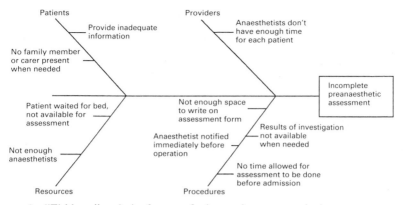

FIG 3—"Fishbone" analysis of reasons for incomplete preanaesthetic assessments.

services could escalate the attention paid to quality by scientifically trained colleagues. Systematic analysis of processes and systems could be useful in identifying where, when, and why things go wrong and could point the way toward changes that should be made. Involving the people who provide or support the service in audit is likely to increase their commitment to improving the service and to lead eventually to benefits to patients as well as staff.

The ultimate power of this approach to quality in healthcare services is in the results of the process of total quality management or continuous quality improvement when all or even most of the individual departments in a healthcare organisation participate in it (box 6).

Box 6 – Outcomes of total quality management

- Development of a shared understanding of practical ways to define and observe quality
- Routine use of scientific methods to measure quality of service throughout the organisation
- A deeper knowledge about how failures in processes and systems can affect outcomes
- Breakdown of traditional organisational barriers and a shift in the organisational attitudes as people learn to identify, communicate with, and respond to their external and internal customers and users
- Measurable improvements in the quality of service to patients

---

1 Secretaries of State for Health, Wales, Northern Ireland, and Scotland. *Working for patients.* London: HMSO, 1989:39–41.
2 Andersen TF, Mooney G. *The challenges of medical practice variations.* Basingstoke: Macmillan Press, 1990.
3 Knaus WA, Draper EA, Wagner DP, Zimmerman JE. An evaluation of outcome from intensive care in major medical centers. *Ann Intern Med* 1986;**104**:410–8.
4 Lembcke PA. Medical auditing by scientific methods. Illustrated by major pelvic surgery. *JAMA* 1956;**162**:645–55.
5 Buckingham WB. Audit – a definition. *QRB* 1975;1:18.
6 Secretaries of State for Health, Wales, Northern Ireland, and Scotland. *Working for patients. Medical audit. Working paper 6.* London: HMSO, 1989.
7 Fowkes FRG. Medical audit cycle: a review of methods and research in clinical practice. *Med Educ* 1982;**16**:228–38.
8 Shaw CD, Costain DW. Guidelines for medical audit: seven principles. *BMJ* 1989;**299**:498–9.
9 Dixon N. *Medical audit primer.* Romsey: Healthcare Quality Quest, 1991.
10 Adapted from Taylor TH, Goldhill DR. *Standards of care in anaesthesia.* Oxford: Butterworth-Heinemann, 1992:14–6,37.
11 Berwick DM. Continuous improvement as an ideal in health care. *N Engl J Med* 1989;**320**:53–6.
12 Berwick DM, Enthoven A, Bunker JP. Quality management in the NHS: the doctor's role – I. *BMJ* 1992;**304**:235–9.
13 Berwick DM, Enthoven A, Bunker JP. Quality management in the NHS: the doctor's role – II. *BMJ* 1992;**304**:304–8.
14 Berwick DM. Heal thyself or heal thy system: can doctors help to improve medical care? *Quality in Health Care* 1992;1(Suppl):S2–8.
15 Pollitt CJ. Audit and accountability: the missing dimension? *J R Soc Med* 1993;**86**:209–11.
16 Donabedian A. *Explorations in quality assessment and monitoring. Vol I. The definition of quality and approaches to its assessment.* Ann Arbor: Health Administration Press, 1980:79–100.
17 Donabedian A. *Explorations in quality assessment and monitoring. Vol I. The definition of quality and approaches to its assessment.* Ann Arbor: Health Administration Press, 1980:129–32.
18 Donabedian A. The assessment of technology and quality. A comparative study of certainties and ambiguities. *Int J Technol Assess Health Care* 1988;**4**:487–96.
19 Luke RD, Boss RW. Barriers limiting the implementation of quality assurance programs. *Health Serv Res* 1981;**16**:305–14.
20 Deming WE. *Out of the crisis.* Cambridge: Massachusetts Institute of Technology Press, 1986.
21 Juran JM, Gryna FM. *Quality planning and analysis.* New York: McGraw-Hill, 1980:1–4.
22 *Total quality management. Part 2. Guide to quality improvement methods. BS 7850: Part 2: 1992.* London: British Standards Institute, 1992.
23 *Quality vocabulary ISO 8402.* Geneva: International Organization for Standardization, 1986.
24 Stebbing L, Dixon N. Meanings of quality in health care. *The Health Summary* 1992;**9**:7–10.
25 Lohr KN, ed. *Medicare. A strategy for quality assurance. Vol I.* Washington DC: National Academy Press, 1990.
26 *Accreditation manual for hospitals.* Oakbrook Terrace IL: Joint Commission on Accreditation of Healthcare Organizations, 1991:260–1.
27 Department of Health. *The quality of medical care. Report of the standing medical advisory committee for the Secretaries of State for Health and Wales.* London: HMSO, 1990.
28 Buck N, Devlin HB, Lunn JN. *The report of a confidential enquiry into perioperative deaths.* London: The Nuffield Provincial Hospitals Trust and The King's Fund, 1989.
29 Cohen MM, Duncan PG, Pope WDB, Biehl D, Tweed WA, MacWilliam L, *et al.* The Canadian four-centre study of anaesthetic outcomes: II. Can outcomes be used to assess the quality of anaesthetic care? *Can J Anaesth* 1992;**39**:430–9.
30 Duncan PG, Cohen MM, Tweed WA, Biehl D, Pope WDB, Merchant RN, *et al.* The Canadian four-centre study of anaesthetic outcomes: III. Are anaesthetic complications predictable in day surgical practice? *Can J Anaesth* 1992;**39**:440–8.
31 Gamil M, Fanning A. The first 24 hours after surgery. *Anaesthesia* 1991;**46**:712–5.

6 Psychology and safety in aviation

JOHN CHAPPELOW

Parallels can be found between any pair of skilled jobs simply because the nature of skills is governed by the underlying characteristics and limitations of humans. For the same reason, any experience in understanding accidents and combating error in one profession may, if studied with appropriate caution, illuminate similar aspects of another. If the investigation and study of error has received more attention in aviation than in anaesthetics, part of the explanation probably lies in the fact that aviation accidents have tended to be more expensive and unavoidably more public than anaesthetic accidents. In presenting some aspects of experience in aviation, I do not intend to suggest that any transfer of wisdom will necessarily be one way, although it is undoubtedly true that anaesthetists have shown a great deal more interest in aviation than pilots have in anaesthetics. Whether this is a difference in breadth of outlook or the relative attractiveness of international flight and major surgery is, perhaps fortunately, beyond the scope of this chapter.

Incidence and types of error

About 40% of serious accidents in the Royal Air Force are ascribed to aircrew error. Other military operators report similar proportions. In the commercial aviation sector various figures have been quoted, some as high as 80%. Comparable statistics in anaesthetics are difficult to obtain, but there are indications that similar proportions hold. Schneider, for example, reported that 92 out of 125 (about 74%) anaesthetic mishaps examined by a Food and Drug Administration panel were associated with operator error.[1] In anaesthetics as in aviation, an enquiry after an accident often faces a difficult question: Why should an experienced, motivated professional, with undoubted skill, make such a mistake? In individual cases the question can seem perplexing. Viewing a large number of such events adds to the confusion. The first step necessary in tackling this problem is to recognise the wide variety of ways in which mistakes come about, and to consider classifying errors according to the characteristic mechanisms involved or the contributory factors. There are several ways of approaching this problem, depending on the degree to which theory or data dictate the classification scheme, and, of course, the theoretical bias of the classifier.

A long term (20 year) study, which is still continuing in the RAF, involves independent investigation by a psychologist of accidents caused by aircrew errors. The results of these investigations are classified according to a scheme which is, as far as possible, data-driven. No particular theoretical view is adopted. The broad findings of the study are shown in Table I. This shows all those factors found to be at least possible contributory causes in more than 10% of the investigations. They are fairly arbitrarily assigned to three broad, common sense categories: predispositions contributed by the aircrew themselves; enabling factors contributed by the organisation, tasks and equipment imposed on aircrew; and what can only be described as immediate causes – the actions, conditions or events that lead directly to an error. Notice that there is no clearly dominant factor. In addition, accidents are usually complex events, so often several factors out of a repertoire of about 40 are cited as contributors. These facts suggest that simple, global remedies will not be found. Reducing the toll of accidents is likely to require a combination of specific remedies targeted at relatively small sub-groups of accidents (improving the conspicuousness of aircraft to reduce mid-air collisions – for example – or modifying a regulation or instruction to avoid ambiguity) and a broad assault designed to improve the routine identification and elimination of risks.

Several of the terms in Table I (for example, disorientation and visual illusion) are clearly peculiar to aviation, or at least unlikely to be relevant to anaesthetic accidents. Several of the larger categories do, however, seem to be potentially relevant. They are personality, life stress, acute (reactive) stress, cognitive failure (a

TABLE I   Factors implicated in errors by air crew

	Percentage
Predisposition	
Personality	22
Inexperience	20
Life stress	14
Enabling factors	
Ergonomics	22
Training/briefing	18
Administration	17
Immediate causes	
Acute stress	25
Cognitive failure	18
Distraction	16
False hypothesis	13
Disorientation	12
Visual illusion	12

mismatch between intentions and actions), and a clutch of enabling factors (ergonomics, training, and administration) which together account for about 40% of accidents caused by aircrew errors. The topics to be considered are, therefore, cognitive function and its limitations, long term predispositions to error, short term factors that degrade performance, and enabling factors that make errors more likely.

Cognitive function and its limitations

The gulf between an expert's and a novice's performance can seem immense. Consider piano playing. While the novice proceeds haltingly, is fully absorbed in the task, and makes frequent errors both in decoding the score and, even when the notes are correctly identified, in hitting the keys, the expert performs fluently on far more demanding pieces, may not even need a score, and concentrates on subtler aspects of interpretation or is capable of holding a conversation at the same time. The novice's mistakes are easy to understand, but inexperience seems (from Table I) not to make a dominating contribution to aircrew error – and this in military aviation, a profession which by its very nature puts large demands on young shoulders. To understand why skilled operators sometimes make mistakes it is first necessary to understand how normal skilled behaviour is achieved, because it seems that errors are a consequence of the normal characteristics of skill and expertise. The cognitive strategies that enable the expert pianist to achieve a polished performance are the same ones that distinguish the captain of an airliner from a trainee pilot. They also form the basis of more common skills that everyone takes for granted, and entail particular risks.

An important feature of human behaviour is that some activities seem to require little or no mental effort, and so can be performed in parallel with other activities. Others seem to absorb all our mental capacity. It is not just a matter of conflicting motor actions; it is a central, mental resource that is implicated. Most adults can ride a bicycle and talk or do mental arithmetic at the same time, but try multiplying two two-digit numbers during a hard fought game of, say, squash or badminton. The unpredictability of the overtly physical game precludes unrelated mental effort. It is also important that activities can be moved from the mentally demanding group to the low-mental-effort group simply by practice; there is no hard and fast categorisation. Indeed a puncture or unexpected obstacle at high speed can suddenly, temporarily reverse the process and change riding a bicycle into the sort of task that excludes all other thought.

Introspection offers an indication of the nature of this limited mental resource. When we perform a difficult or novel task, what it demands is our attention; the task becomes the principal thing of which we are conscious. And attention seems to be flexible, both in terms of the sensory modalities to which it refers, and temporally. The contents of consciousness need not be the results of current stimulation; they can be formed from memories of past events, or imaginative constructions. Attention has the character of memory for the present. It enables information of present interest, from a variety of sources, to be held in consciousness while it is evaluated or used in decision making or computation.

There is good experimental evidence for this separate, short term form of memory. Indeed, three qualitatively different types of memory store have been identified: short term or working memory, long term memory, and sensory stores. They differ in terms of capacity, the duration of storage, and the mechanisms involved in forgetting.

Working memory

Working memory seems to have three components. The best

understood, known as the articulatory loop, handles phonological (speech based) information. Its capacity is limited to only a few items – about enough for a telephone number – and decay takes only a few seconds. The memory can, however, be maintained indefinitely by rehearsal using articulatory processes connected with speech. There seems to be an independent but structurally similar component used for storing spatial information. Like the articulatory loop it involves a passive information store and an active rehearsal mechanism, in this case possibly based on the system that controls eye movements.

The least well understood component of working memory is known as the central executive. It is thought to be capable of handling any type of information, and to be responsible for the integration of information from disparate sources as well as scheduling the allocation of mental resources. Its capacity is thought to be limited, but has so far defied measurement. The central executive's rather grand title reflects the importance attached to its functions. It has also been aptly described by Baddeley as an "area of residual ignorance."[2] It is, perhaps, inevitable that all the (so far) experimentally inaccessible functions of working memory should seem to reside in one enigmatic block. If any progress can be made in this area, a more complex, but also more satisfying picture should emerge. For the moment some important features of working memory are clear: although both spatial and phonological information can be stored, the overall capacity is limited and maintaining the memory for more than a few seconds demands effort and consumes precious resources. Information in working memory is also vulnerable to interference from new inputs. These limitations demand effort-saving strategies in gathering information from the world and controlling our actions.

Long term memory

In contrast to working memory, long term memory seems to have an enormous capacity, and to store information indefinitely. We are aware of this information, however, only when it is transferred to working memory. Long term memory also seems to involve several sub-systems, but the distinctions involved are not always clearly drawn. For example, it is clear that some of the information in long term memory can be described as semantic. It involves knowledge about the world: Julius Caesar was a Roman, the tyre pressures on my car are 32 psi (front) and 30 psi (rear), and

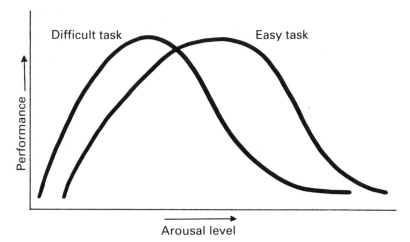

FIG 1—The Yerkes-Dodson law

so on. Other information is best described as episodic. It relates to my own personal experience. It is not clear, however, that different processes are involved in forming these two types of memory, and sometimes the distinction between them is difficult to make. For example, recalling the tyre pressures also brings to mind incidents involving flat tyres and any episodic recall also entails semantic knowledge. It is interesting that interviewing survivors of accidents often shows an apparent change in the way that the story is told after several repetitions from a detailed, possibly confused, pattern that seems to invoke actual impressions of the event, to a more coherent, sparser account that is often less informative (and sometimes at variance with other evidence). This may reflect a change in the way the information is stored, semantic coding being more economical. The change that takes place in fishermen's tales with retelling probably involves a similar shift in balance between the more veridical episodic encoding and the more "meaningful" semantic encoding.

Another useful distinction is between declarative knowledge (which embraces both semantic and episodic memory) and procedural knowledge. Procedural knowledge is of particular interest in the context of error because it involves the mechanisms that control or guide performance of a task without reference to underlying factual knowledge. Knowing how to ride a bicycle is a good example of procedural knowledge. Once attained, the knowledge persists indefinitely, and is instantly available should the opportunity to exercise it arise. It is also peculiarly difficult to communicate the fundamentals of the skill verbally. This last point is not true of all procedural knowledge, however, and the distinction from declarative knowledge is not entirely clear cut. In the context of error analysis some – Reason and Mycielska, for example – have found it useful to classify tasks according to the type of knowledge involved in their execution.[3] The most automatic activities are described as skill-based; they demand little conscious attention, and verbalisation of the processes involved may be difficult. Rule-based behaviour involves more easily described procedures, for example "i" before "e" except after "c"; to change a wheel, first loosen the wheel nuts, then jack up the car, remove the nuts, and wheel, then reverse the process with the new wheel. It demands a little more conscious monitoring if actions are to be performed in the right order without omissions. The most demanding activities are described as knowledge-based. Here the activity is largely unautomatic, the mental load is considerable, and artificial memory aids may be required, for example check lists, computational notes, diagrams, and maps.

Again it is often difficult, if not impossible, to make precise distinctions in practical cases. Most complex tasks involve more or less unconscious procedural elements and overall strategies based on explicitly definable knowledge. With increasing experience, the trainee's behaviour on some aspects of his tasks might be said to progress from one level to the next as less and less conscious attention is required. This is surely not a general description of acquisition of the skills or expertise, however. It is, for example, possible to describe the sequence of actions involved in changing gear in a car. Some people are even capable of explaining in detail the mechanical consequences of these control movements. For most people, however, gear changing is simply a "knack"; attempting to convey it in words to a learner driver can be almost pointless. With a little practice, however, the knack is acquired – whether or not the learner understands the mechanical details. Nevertheless, the distinction between skill, rule, and knowledge-based behaviours does have the merit of reflecting an important descriptor of a task in the degree of conscious attention it demands of the operator. It is interesting that errors in knowledge-based behaviour are not listed as immediate causes in Table I, but cognitive failures are well represented. Cognitive failures involve a mismatch between intentions and actions. The correct drill is selected, but items are omitted, confused with others from a similar drill, or operated in reverse (raising rather than lowering a lever). Cognitive failures are often associated with distractions or preoccupation in otherwise normal and undemanding circumstances. When knowledge-based errors are identified in an investigation, they are often associated with failures in training or briefing, or the administrative background (which includes the framing of orders, manuals, and instructions).

Can this be taken as guidance for the likely pattern of errors in other professions? Probably not entirely. The data on aircrew errors do point to cognitive failure as an important area of vulnerability in skilled performance, which is certainly not confined to aviation. It is true, however, that aviation, and military aviation in particular, involves highly standardised routines and rituals which are designed to minimise the workload entailed in knowledge-based performance. Such a strategy promises a high probability of success in extremely demanding missions, without raising personnel selection criteria to unrealistic levels. It also necessarily biases the type of error likely to predominate in any collection of accident investigations.

Sensory stores

Little of the information available at any moment in the sensory domain is allowed into the focus of attention. But that focus can shift quickly – from reading this text to sounds coming from another room, say, or the sensations produced as your hands support the book. When the impetus for a shift of attention is produced by an unexpected external event, such as your own name cropping up in the conversation in the next room, some antecedents of that stimulus (the beginning of the sentence, for example) may also be noticed. Experimental evidence suggests that this remarkable, and useful, feat is not achieved through prescience, but by routine, short term, storage of sensory information. Sensory stores seem to have unlimited capacity, but retain information for, at most, a second or so. This allows not only selection of the information to be processed, but also some interpretation on the basis of past experience and current context.

Perception is, therefore, in part driven by expectation. This is a labour-saving ruse that takes advantage of redundancy and predictability in the real world in constructing a representation of it.

The written word is particularly redundant, as this sentence about a tailoring deficiency shows: "Th# sl##v#s #f th# sh#rt w#r# a l#ttl# t## sh#rt." Despite the lack of vowels, it is unlikely to take much longer to decipher this sentence than it would normally. And the interpretation of "sh#rt" should change naturally with context. The advantages of this system are considerable: it reduces the resources required to interpret the world, and allows some flexibility in selection and interpretation based on succeeding as well as preceding information.

The disadvantage is, of course, a risk of misperception or misinterpretation by too great a reliance on previous experience and present expectations. In Table I these errors are listed in the false hypothesis category. Often they are associated with a preceding cognitive failure. The pilot is distracted or preoccupied during his prelanding checks. The checks, which he has done so often that he hardly need think about them, are completed, but with an omission. He "knows" he has lowered the undercarriage, so a routine glance at the undercarriage indicator gives the expected result, not the true state of affairs, and the landing continues without wheels. Even after landing, the pilot may not correctly diagnose the cause of the strange noises and bumps as the aircraft slides down the runway, so strong is his expectation.

Overview

The system described above is flexible and efficient. In familiar situations the effort required is minimised; well practised routines and rules of thumb operate almost automatically, and the signals required to direct actions or initiate new responses are selected without much deliberation. In taxing or problematical situations a more effort-intensive approach can be adopted. The environment is scanned for the signs that identify the problem or situation; previously effective solutions are recalled from past experience and implemented. When the situation is novel, a deliberate, more or less systematic exercise in information gathering and conceptual reasoning may be required. The expert approaches his task with all three strategies at his disposal. Long-term goals may be consciously set, and these define the skills required and the experience he will have to draw on in executing his shorter-term plans.

The weaknesses of the system are characteristic of the resources deployed in each type of approach. The capacity of working memory is an all too evident limit on efficiency in conceptual reasoning. When diagnosis and response are required in a fairly short time, and aides memoires are not available, then it is common that some relevant information is overlooked or given insufficient weight, particularly if it does not fit the first tenable hypothesis that comes to mind. Solutions may be proposed that are focused on the observable symptoms, but without thought for possible side-effects of the solutions (a trivial example is replacing a blown fuse with one of higher rating). When there is just too much to think about, there is a strong temptation to test hypotheses in a concrete manner without considering the possible consequences of the intervention. In more routine circumstances, minor slips and lapses are more likely. Monitoring may fail to detect the signs; the situation is seen as normal – as expected. About two thirds of the cognitive failures reported in Table I happened in routine, undemanding circumstances. Often all that was required was a minor distraction. The consequences seem out of proportion to the precipitating event. It is an important finding for any safety oriented occupation that normal behaviour in normal circumstances carries an appreciable risk of serious error.

Factors affecting performance

Military aircrew have to contend with various environmental stressors not commonly encountered in the operating theatre: heat, vibration, noise, and acceleration are all catered for with special equipment. Other stressors occur in both anaesthetics and aviation. The most obvious is the acute, reactive stress associated with life-threatening emergencies. The fact that the pilot's life is among those threatened, whereas the anaesthetist's is not, is probably not an important difference.

The effects of stressors on performance are complex and varied. To some extent the concept of arousal simplifies (perhaps oversimplifies) discussion of these effects. It implies a continuum of activation from extreme drowsiness to extreme excitement. Psychological indicators of arousal level include alertness, sensitivity to stimulation, and performance on tests. Physiological indicators, such as heart rate and skin resistance, sometimes, but only sometimes, show useful correlations with psychological variables. Figure 1 embodies two ideas which have proved a useful, if incomplete, description of the relationship between arousal level and performance for many years.[4] The first idea is that there is an optimum arousal level for any task. This implies an inverted "U" relationship with performance. This is a difficult hypothesis to test experimentally, of course. The second idea is that easy tasks are more tolerant of high arousal levels than difficult ones. Level of difficulty in this context obviously depends on the training and experience of the operator. Further individual differences (see the section on personality) also complicate the picture. Variations in arousal level seem to affect performance largely by changing attentional capacity and processing speed. To some extent these changes are moderated by learned strategies in the control of attention.

At low levels of arousal, such as might occur after a long period of work at night, particularly if the work is unstimulating or monotonous, responses take longer and lapses of attention and omissions are more likely to occur. Given noise, stimulants (such as caffeine or interesting conversation), or sufficient motivation, apparently normal levels of efficiency can be achieved – though the less important tasks may be neglected.

Fatigue and sleep deprivation are common stressors, but they do not figure in Table I. This is not to suggest that they never contribute to aircrew error, but the evidence is that they make only a minor contribution. In civil aviation, some of which routinely involves long periods on duty, time zone shifts, and disruption of circadian rhythms, there may be more scope for fatigue and sleep deprivation to affect performance. In both the military and civilian sectors, however, duty cycles and rest periods are governed by firm regulation and are closely monitored.

At high levels of arousal, such as might be provoked by an emergency, information may be processed more quickly but at the expense of a reduction in the capacity of working memory. Control of attention becomes more of a problem. The reduction in capacity of working memory can be compensated for by increased attentional selectivity – focusing intently on the important information – but impairment of perceptual discrimination may allow superficially relevant stimuli to become distracting, so disrupting performance.

Acute reactive stress

The errors coded under "acute stress" in Table I were mainly caused by mechanical problems – for example, engine fires or bird strikes. A few were the result of previous mishandling by the pilot, or disorientation. The main category of problems generated (about 30%) are best described as a disorganisation of response: the wrong drills were selected, or the pilot's analysis of the emergency was haphazard and ineffective. Slow responses and precipitate action were about equally likely (about 10% of the total each), and narrowing of attention and cognitive failure together accounted for another 30% of the cases.

There is no reason to suppose that this pattern is in any way unusual, nor likely to be representative of that found in non-aviation emergencies. Extremely detailed knowledge of the job, the emergency, and the operator would be required to predict the type of failure to be expected. Some general guidance on the operator's contribution is given in the section on predisposition.

Predisposition

State: life stress

A popular lay explanation for pilot error involves domestic and other pressures. The association between stressful life events (both positive and negative) and heart disease and other illnesses is well known. A similar statistical association between the incidence of life events and involvement in flying accidents has been reported at least once, but this is clearly a difficult area for research, and further analysis can suggest other interpretations.[56] Close examination of the accidents coded in Table I under "life stress" shows at most only two cases in which a link with life events can confidently be averred. Both were rather special cases, and did not involve a general depletion of the pilots' ability to cope with the stresses of work.

It is possible that military aviation allows greater compartmentalisation than some other professions. The crew are isolated from other distractions and pressures while performing the task, and, in many cases, the critical parts of the task (while airborne) last for relatively short periods. Many people can cope under these circumstances, unless the stress is causing noticeable sleep disruption. It is also likely that individual differences play a large part in regulating the impact of life events.

Trait: personality

The scientific description of personality can be approached in various ways. Two dimensions that have proved useful in many fields of investigation are extraversion and neuroticism.[7] Questionnaire tests of extraversion and neuroticism distinguish different types of deviant personality and psychiatric disorder, and also show reliable differences between professional groups. In addition, scores on such tests account for some of the variation in the way people approach tasks, cope with a range of stressors, and behave generally. Extraverts are assumed to require more stimulation than introverts to excite the central nervous system. As a result, extraverts are active, sociable, and impulsive, while introverts are passive, reserved, and thoughtful. A high neuroticism score indicates a labile autonomic nervous system; it would be associated with an emotional or moody disposition. A low score would indicate stability.

Introverts tend to work in a methodical manner, and hence to be slower than extraverts, who may make more mistakes in the interests of speed. Stimulants and threatening circumstances, by raising arousal level, would tend to be detrimental for introverts (by overarousal), but may improve extraverts' performance, as they tend to be chronically underaroused. The introvert performs better, however, when sustained vigilance is required.

A high neuroticism score has implications for performance in threatening circumstances. Anxiety may divert mental resources into unproductive worry and so degrade performance. Psychosomatic illness can result from prolonged exposure to such stress. A high score may also accentuate the differences between introverts and extraverts in terms of liability to accidents.

Several studies in aviation and road safety have implicated neuroticism or some form of maladjustment. High extraversion scores have also been found to be associated with involvement in accidents. Contradictory findings and failures to find any association are by no means unknown, however, and it is not possible to claim that a clear picture has emerged. Bearing in mind that not all accidents are likely to involve an important contribution from personality variables, it is obvious that large numbers would be needed to establish any correlations. It is also likely that some attention should be given to classifying types of accident (further increasing the numbers required).

Table I shows that about 22% of accidents caused by aircrew error in the RAF have a possible association with personality. It has been possible to classify about two thirds of these on the basis of descriptors used in personal records. Two groups have emerged.

One is described as underconfident, nervous, or prone to over-react; the other as overconfident, reckless, and heedless of rules. It is tempting to apply the labels "unstable introvert" and "unstable extravert" respectively, but more evidence is required. It is clear, however, that one group (the first) tends to be associated with accidents involving mishandled emergencies, and the other with accidents involving unauthorised or risky manoeuvres, or failure to appreciate risk.

Parallels probably exist in many other professions. Even if "joy riding" is not possible, there is always some scope for ill-considered experimentation, corner-cutting, and, of course, mishandling of emergencies. It is also clear that future research should not be expected to produce simple correlations between personality measures and accident involvement. It would be wise to expect a bipolar relationship with extraversion mediated by neuroticism, and to classify accidents according to the types of error involved. Personality tests can provide some guidance in selecting aircrew, and are used by many airlines. They are, however, relatively imprecise instruments, and their usefulness in selection obviously depends on the ratio of suitable candidates to vacant posts. In most contexts differences in personality remain a management issue.

Trait: cognitive function

In addition, individual differences in cognitive functioning may play a part in liability to accidents. Broadbent *et al* suggested that the ability to cope with chronic, mild stress, and liability to cognitive error may both be related to stable biases in cognitive style, those with a more obsessional style being less vulnerable to stress and less prone to cognitive failure. They also suggested that under stress cognitive styles may become more extreme.[8] Cognitive style may therefore identify those who are vulnerable to life stress and even, possibly, mediate a relationship between life stress and accident involvement.

Enabling factors

The first three enabling factors listed in Table I together account for about 40% of the accidents conventionally described as caused by "aircrew error." The potential for such system-induced errors increases with the sophistication and power of the systems used. Aviators and anaesthetists both increasingly rely on indirect apprehension of important data and indirect control of the system. There are obvious benefits in the use of technology to supplement human capabilities, but the designer of equipment faces real challenges in devising suitable interfaces. Conflicting requirements have to be met. Both the novice and the expert require easily interpretable displays and accessible, simple controls. The expert, however, may require more detailed information, or a more flexible operating style than the novice. Ease of operation in controls is obviously desirable, but may facilitate mis-selections. In addition, the training and administrative background set the context in which the operator works, and both can easily provide opportunities for misinformation and confusion.

The variety of enabling factors is enormous. One unifying aspect is the fact that such problems are identifiable before they cause an accident, and, in contrast to most of the psychological factors discussed above, are in principle amenable to relatively simple remedies. The inquiries into many major disasters (Chernobyl, Challenger, the Herald of Free Enterprise) have provided examples. The failure of senior management to remedy this type of problem may result from lack of imagination, error of judgement, or an unfortunate ordering of priorities. The failure of professionals operating the system to demand action may be caused by a perceived lack of influence or, perversely, an aspect of the "professional" attitude. Professionals expect to be able to cope. Performing under less than optimum conditions does afford some satisfaction. Complaining about inadequate equipment, or questioning common practice may seem "unprofessional," particularly if it involves an admission that something is not understood. In both military and civilian aviation steps have been taken to circumvent this problem, and these are dealt with below.

Remedies

The picture of the human presented above looks somewhat discouraging. Although capable of acquiring complex skills and of retaining large amounts of knowledge, he is likely to fail in a number of ways. If the task is unusually demanding or the context too stressful, his behaviour is likely to become disorganised, skills may break down, information may well be overlooked, disregarded, or improperly interpreted; if things are going well, and the task demands are slight, the experienced operator may fail to execute "simple" procedures properly, or become inattentive. Depending on his personality, he may tolerate stress only poorly, or impulsively deviate from standard practice. Some of these problems are relatively intractable features of human nature. Long term research may eventually provide palliatives. But our perspective so far has been exclusively error-oriented. It is as well to bear in mind that, in contrast to the situation in experimental studies, it is not unusual for many hours of successful performance to separate errors in real tasks, and humans do routinely identify and correct slips, lapses, and misunderstandings. The very rarity of error makes applied research and planning for practical remedial action difficult. Nevertheless, proactive remedial action is possible. Three major features of proactive effort in aviation are standardisation, simulation, and competency checks.

Standardisation applies to all aspects of aviation. As far as possible all the equipment fitted to a fleet of aircraft will conform to a common standard, and to some extent common standards are applied across fleets. There are economic reasons for this approach, but safety advantages accrue as well. More importantly, standard operating procedures are defined according to the best available advice and experience. This ensures that crews who have never met before can work together efficiently and safely, and that the best practice is applied universally. When flaws in the design of equipment or procedures do come to light, again remedies can be applied universally; the number and variety of risks latent in the system is minimised.

An advantage of standardisation is the criteria it provides against which to judge performance. Aircrew are routinely assessed for basic skills and for their ability to cope with emergencies. A standard set of emergencies is defined (for example engine failure during take-off), and the crew members have to demonstrate their ability to handle these emergencies at regular intervals. The procedures under which these skills are assessed are themselves monitored and standardised by independent authorities.

Simulation has provided the means of testing skills in emergencies safely, and more effectively. The technology used in flight simulators can support effective assessment and instruction through the use of replays, and graphical records. Regular simulator training in emergencies, besides ensuring competence in handling the most likely and most threatening mishaps, also increases the crew's general confidence, and may make them more resistant to the stress of unexpected problems. In addition, simulators are increasingly being used to support special courses designed to make aircrew aware of human factors issues and, in particular, the effective use of resources, both material and human. A prominent element of many such courses is guidance in interpersonal relations and successful cooperation among crew members.

The management of any modern flying enterprise necessarily involves consideration of safety issues. Not only accidents, but also minor incidents are investigated thoroughly. The lessons learned are fed back into operational practice through flight safety organisations that permeate almost every level of the management structure. These organisations also seek out hazards through flight safety inspections or routine monitoring of the records made by airborne data recorders. Such measures obviously have to be applied with a degree of tact and sympathy, if the cooperation of the operators is to be maintained.

In addition to the schemes for compulsory reporting of incidents, both military and civilian operators also have confidential reporting systems. Again there is potential for unnecessary embarrassment or mistrust, but, with care, such schemes do provide valuable information, and, obviously, have the potential to prevent accidents.

Conclusions

Many of the most important errors derive directly from normal characteristics of human skilled behaviour. General principles on how to cater for this vulnerability are by no means established, but recognising the fact has, at least, moved the debate on in aviation from issues of blame to research issues and possible remedy. In general, by relying on standardised procedures, aviation seems to have reduced the potential for errors in knowledge-based activity; as a result the predominant, primary, immediate cause of aircrew error seems to be cognitive failure.

There is some evidence suggesting that personality may predispose some individuals to a particular type of risk. Many airlines use personality tests in their selection procedures. Such tools obviously provide only guidance rather than identification, and their use in a selection process inevitably depends on the ratio of high quality candidates to vacant posts.

The stress caused by emergencies does contribute to aircrew

error, but regular simulator training, and competency checks, serve to reduce its impact. The role of domestic stress is best described as undecided. The nature of the (particularly military) aviation task may provide a measure of protection. Many other stresses associated with flying are routinely contained. Fatigue may in general be counted among these because of regulation and monitoring.

Aviation has in large measure embraced a safety oriented culture. Standardisation, simulation, and competency checks are entrenched in the system, and serve to limit the potential for risk and its impact. In addition, there is an active interest in identifying risks through inspection, investigation, and incident reporting schemes.

It is undoubtedly true that there are parallels with all these factors in anaesthetics. The success of the aviation industry in reducing the accident rate to its present low level may encourage further parallel development.

1 Schneider AJL. Regulation of anaesthesia devices in the USA. *Baillière's Clinical Anaesthesiology* 1988;2:353–66.
2 Baddeley A. *Working memory*. Oxford: Clarendon Press, 1986.
3 Reason J, Mycielska JD. *Absent minded?* Englewood Cliffs: Prentice Hall, 1982.
4 Yerkes RM, Dodson JD. The relation of strength of stimulus to rapidity of habit formation. *Journal of ComparativeNeurology and Pyschology* 1908;18:459–82.
5 Alkov RA, Borowsky MS. A questionnaire study of psychological background factors in US Navy aircraft accidents. *Aviat Space Environ Med* 1980;51:860–3.
6 Alkov RA, Borowsky MS, Gaynor JA. Stress coping and the US Navy aircrew factor mishap. *Aviat Space Environ Med* 1982;53:1112–5.
7 Eysenck HJ, Eysenck SBG. *Manual of the Eysenck personality inventory*. Sevenoaks: Hodder and Stoughton, 1964.
8 Broadbent DE, Broadbent MHP, Jones JL. Performance correlates of self-reported cognitive failure and obsessionality. *Br J Clin Psychol* 1986;25:285–99.

7 Critical incidents in anaesthesia

M CLARE DERRINGTON

The critical incident technique is a process developed by psychologists to evaluate aspects of human behaviour and to study the causes of good and poor performance. It has been interpreted and applied in anaesthetic practice for some years. Cooper *et al* used it to investigate the factors that predisposed anaesthetists to make mistakes and to identify circumstances which encouraged error.[1] They collected factual accounts of anaesthetic problems or potential problems. Data were excluded if neither human error nor equipment failure featured. A total of 82% of the incidents that they collected resulted from human error and 14% from failure of equipment; 4% were unaccounted for as they did not fit easily into either category. The findings of that study have been misquoted widely as evidence for the "fact" that 82% of mishaps or potential mishaps in anaesthetic practice are the result of human error.[2-5] If incidents that resulted neither from human error nor equipment failure are automatically discarded by the study protocol then the results of the study are biased and such conclusions cannot be drawn.

There is also a misconception among anaesthetists about the origin of the term "critical incident" and its meaning has been misinterpreted to mean "anaesthetic hazard" or "potential hazard."[6] To be strictly correct, a critical incident has to be defined in the context of a study, whether it is of preventable anaesthetic mishaps,[1] the evaluation of flying skill,[7] or the ability of anaesthetists to give epidural anaesthetics.[8]

Though there have been flaws in the interpretation of the term, adaptations of the critical incident technique have been used to improve equipment design and develop protocols in anaesthetic practice which have proved to be valuable. In many cases, however, too narrow an interpretation of the procedure has limited the extent of its use. A full examination of the technique as it is used in psychology will show that it could be more widely used to improve quality and safety in anaesthesia.

Development of the technique

In 1954 Flanagan, a psychologist, wrote a paper in which he described the critical incident technique, which he had been working with for some years.[9] He presented it as an objective scientific method of studying human behaviour. It had been applied in the United States Army Air Force during the second world war. Much attention had been focused on selecting recruits for the Air Force who had the appropriate skills to become good pilots. The reasons given for expulsion from flight training school were, however, often too vague to apply as selection criteria for new pilots. To obtain more objective information the trainers were asked to give an account of factual incidents that described the successful performance of pilots and others which showed inadequate performance. These were then analysed and used for the recruitment of suitable candidates.

Using similar methods the reasons for the failure of bombing missions, the best characteristics for combat leadership, and the causes of disorientation while flying, were also investigated. The results of these studies initiated changes in selection and training procedures and in the layout of cockpits and instruments. The method – subsequently known as *the critical incident technique* – could be used to measure performance or proficiency, to make observations about job design and training, or to assess operating procedures and the design of equipment.

Instead of formulating opinions, interpretations, and hunches about an activity or subject, trained observers collect large numbers of factual observations which make an important positive or negative contribution to the activity being studied. When these critical incidents are analysed and categorised they indicate the requirements of a particular subject or activity with objectivity and precision; these are the *critical requirements* of the activity, those which are important in determining its success or failure.

106

Definitions

An incident is any observable human activity that is sufficiently complete in itself to permit inferences and predictions to be made about the person performing the act.

A critical incident is an incident the purpose or intent of which seems fairly clear to the observer and the consequences of which are sufficiently definite to leave little doubt about its effect.

There is no single rigid set of rules governing the collection of data. The critical incident technique is a flexible set of principles that have to be modified and adapted to apply to the particular situation under study.

Designing a study

The five stages of designing a critical incident study are shown in box 1.

Box 1 – Design of a critical incident study

- Description of general aim of activity under study
- Specification of: Observers
  Groups to be observed
  Observations to be made
- Collection of data
- Analysis of data
- Interpretation and reporting of data

The first step is to define the aim of the activity to be studied. Usually there is not one general aim and there is rarely one person or group who constitute an absolute authoritative source about the aim. For example, a patient, a surgeon, a theatre sister, and a hospital manager might all define the aim of the anaesthetist's job differently. The definition of the purpose of the activity is important and several authorities should be consulted.

The next step is to decide on who should collect the data and what level of training is required of them, so that the data that they collect are relevant. The data are usually collected by investigators trained in interviewing and the collection of information who have been given a brief introduction to the topic being studied. They

107

have to be clear exactly what the aims of the study are, who they are studying, and the sort of activities that they should report.

Methods by which the data can be collected are shown in box 2.

Box 2 – Methods of collecting data

- By interview, after an explanation, the subject is asked to recall relevant events. In some studies group interviews are conducted, which are less time consuming
- Questionnaire forms (use fewer resources)
- Record forms may be completed by trained observers as events occur or the study group can telephone to report incidents immediately after they have happened – prospective critical incident survey

---

The anonymity of both the reporter and the subject is important to encourage accuracy and objectivity, particularly when ineffective behaviour is being reported. A clear description of the event also suggests accuracy.

The number of critical incidents required to obtain a useful result depends on the complexity of the activity being studied and may be as many as several thousand. To ensure comprehensive data two tests can be applied. When the addition of a hundred new critical incidents adds only two or three new categories to the pool existing data are probably adequate, and it is important to have at least three examples of each category of critical incident.

If the sample is representative, the observers well qualified, the judgements appropriate and well defined, and the procedures for reporting accurate, the stated requirements can be expected to be comprehensive, detailed, and valid. The purpose of analysing data is to summarise them efficiently so they may be used easily. Classification can be according to use – for example, in training or for the selection of suitable people for a job. Categorisation of data is subjective and should be checked by several authorities.

Validation of data

The reliability and validity of the critical incident technique was confirmed by Anderson and Nilsson who investigated job and training requirements of store managers in Swedish groceries.[10] Store managers' superiors, store managers themselves, assistants, and customers were interviewed and nearly 2000 critical incidents were collected. A critical incident was defined as an account of the behaviour of a store manager that indicated that he was either particularly good or particularly bad at being a store manager. When two thirds of the incidents had been classified, 95% of the subcategories had already appeared, which indicated that the data were fairly complete.

The structure of the material obtained by the different interviewers was similar on analysis and 24 psychology students were asked to recategorise 100 of the critical incidents chosen at random. The category system was found to be plausible and not too subjective. The validity of the study was then tested in two ways. First the training literature for the job of store manager was analysed and fitted into the category system of the study, and secondly the subcategories were rated by 300 people – superiors, store managers, and psychology students. The authors concluded that the information collected by the critical incident technique was both reliable and valid.

Applications of the technique

The critical incident technique has been applied with great success to defining job requirements[11] and the selection of foremen and supervisors.[12] After the war the University of Pittsburgh was inundated with applications to the dental school. The critical incident technique was applied to the prediction of performance of dental students and the results of the study enabled the establishment of criteria for use in the selection of suitable candidates.[13] Critical incident techniques were applied in medicine for the first time to investigate the type and cause of errors in the giving of drugs by nursing staff.[14]

The method was later applied to the investigation of patient care by physicians, surgeons, paediatricians and obstetricians,[15] and later still in the analysis of professional behaviour of various doctors in child health to elucidate the skills required.[16] In this latter study critical incidents reports were collected from general practitioners, paediatricians, parents, health visitors, community doctors, and pharmacists. They were asked to recall occasions when they had seen what seemed to them to be examples of particularly good or poor professional practice of doctors working in child health. The author felt that the technique "though time consuming both in the collection of incidents and their analysis, provides objective data on the requirements of good medical practice in a way which is unmatched by any other method."

Cooper's model of critical incident collection in anaesthesia

Cooper *et al* were the first anaesthetists to apply critical incident analysis to anaesthetic practice. Blum suggested that it might be of value in relationship to the design of anaesthetic equipment: "It is time for the anesthesiologist to realise that human perception and reaction can influence the effectiveness of his equipment, and to recognise that appropriate guidelines can assure the most fundamental form of safeguard."[17]

In their first study, Cooper *et al* set out to examine errors and equipment failures in anaesthetic practice. They redefined the components of the critical incident technique in the framework of anaesthetic practice and in the context of what they wanted to investigate. Their definition of a critical incident (together with those of others) is given in box 3.

By including descriptions of events during which there was no morbidity or mortality (though there might have been if someone had not taken action) they hoped to establish a much wider database for formulating and evaluating hypotheses about the aetiology of anaesthetic errors. They felt that anonymous reporting would encourage frank, honest accounts of mistakes that had been made and they also asked for information about any *"associated factors"* which they defined as conditions at the time of a critical incident that might have predisposed to the development of the incident or hindered its prompt detection.

Box 3 – Definitions of critical incidents from different studies

Cooper et al,[1 18–20 22] *Williamson,*[29 30] and *Runciman*[31]
- A critical incident is an occurrence that could have led (if not discovered or corrected in time) or did lead to an undesirable outcome ranging from increased length of hospital stay to death. It must also involve error by a member of the anaesthetic team or a failure of the anaesthetists' equipment to function; occur while

---

the patient is under anaesthetic care; be described in clear detail by an observer or member of the anaesthetic team; and be clearly preventable

Craig and *Wilson*[23]
- Any anaesthetic mishap, major or minor, which was harmful or potentially harmful to the patient and associated with human error or failure of equipment

Currie et al[24] *(critical events)*
- To collect prospectively, non-anecdotal data on any event associated with anaesthesia (general, regional, or local) which had the potential to result in an adverse outcome irrespective of whether or not any adverse sequelae were noted (four events were excluded from their analysis because they were considered unpreventable – so this must also have been in the definition albeit tacitly)

Currie[25] *(critical event)*
- Any untoward and preventable mishap which was associated with general or regional anaesthesia which led, or could have led, to an undesirable outcome

Kumar et al[26]
- An incident or mistake which could be harmful or potentially harmful to the patient during the management of anaesthesia

Short et al[28]
- An incident that affected or could have affected the safety of the patient whilst under the care of the anaesthetist

Galletly and *Mushet*[27] *(anaesthesia system error)*
- Inappropriate or undesirable performance of people or equipment which was unanticipated and which reduced, or had the potential for reducing, effectiveness, safety, or system performance

McKay and *Noble*[32]
- A critical incident was recorded by the investigator if an unexpected physiological change severe enough to require intervention by the anaesthetist to prevent a likely adverse outcome was signalled first by the oximeter

Vaughan et al[34] *(Anaesthesia related consequence)*
- Pivotal occurrences requiring physician or nursing intervention that could lead, if not discovered or corrected in time, to an undesirable outcome

Cooper et al[33] *(recovery room impact event)*
- An unanticipated, undesirable, possibly anaesthesia-related effect that required intervention, was pertinent to recovery room care, and did or could cause mortality or at least moderate morbidity

Their first paper presented data from interviews with anaesthetic personnel in a large teaching hospital.[1] The interviewer had wide professional experience of the interview technique and had received a brief introduction to anaesthesia. The subjects who were interviewed, all of whom were anaesthetists, were asked to describe preventable happenings that they had observed involving either equipment failure or human error and to specify any associated circumstances. Twenty five pilot interviews were conducted to establish the technique and methods of categorisation of data, and then 47 further interviews took place. The interviews lasted from 60 to 90 minutes. The average number of incidents recounted was seven for staff anaesthetists and eight for trainees though there was a wide variation.

Of the incidents reported, a fifth had occurred more than three years previously and just over half within the last year. The incidents were categorised and the most common were reported together with associated factors. The study differed from many of the later critical incident studies in that no firm definition of an acceptable critical incident was given to the interviewees and no specific types of incidents were suggested. The data were included only if they fitted in with their definition of a critical incident. The most frequent events included breathing circuit disconnections, inadvertent gas flow changes, confusion with syringes, problems with gas supply and disconnection of intravenous lines. "Associated factors" included inadequate experience and unfamiliarity with equipment, poor communication, haste, inattention, carelessness, fatigue, and failure to perform a normal check of equipment.

They then extended their database to include a total of 1089 events. Some of these data were collected prospectively; subjects were asked to telephone as soon as possible after the "critical incident" to report the details. In subsequent papers the group highlighted various circumstances including the relief of one anaesthetist by another and its effect on the discovery or generation of untoward events (*relief associated phenomena*).[18] They produced a specific analysis of those mishaps which resulted in harm to patients (*substantive negative outcomes*),[19] and they also used their data to evaluate the effectiveness of some monitoring devices.[20]

Their data can be criticised because they included events recalled from more than three years before the interview. Allnutt reviewed human factors in accidents and described work from psychologists and experts in accident investigation who had found that as time after an event increased the account became clearer and simpler: "From the moment an aircraft crashes, or an accident occurs in the operating theatre, one of the two major sources of evidence starts to decay rapidly and to become distorted. This source is the memory of the participants, both direct and indirect for the event. A large amount of laboratory and anecdotal evidence shows that memory decreases rapidly over time and that it is distorted in the direction of simplicity and coherence".[21] Cooper *et al* later described a qualitative difference in their critical incidents when they were collected prospectively rather than retrospectively. More equipment failures were reported in the prospective group,[19] and they postulated that this was because people had a more lasting memory of their own mistakes as opposed to failure of equipment that occurred during their practice.

Despite the criticisms, Cooper *et al* introduced a much needed method of assessment of anaesthetic working practices which could be carried out constructively to improve safety and the quality of care. The results of their early work were probably instrumental in causing the widespread adoption of low pressure alarms in the breathing circuit during the mechanical ventilation of a paralysed patient. "This kind of analysis identifies acute problems that require action. At the very least, all mechanical ventilators used during anesthesia should give some obvious indication of a breathing circuit disconnection".[22]

Other workers

The methods of Cooper's group were quickly adopted by other workers in departmental[23-28] and multicentre investigations,[29] and there were soon proposals to do the same nationally and internationally.[30 31] In most cases the data in these later studies were collected prospectively on questionnaire and report forms. Many of the "critical incidents" and their "associated factors" are similar despite quite variable definitions of the data to be collected (box 3). This list also contains definitions from a study investigating the role of pulse oximetry[32] and of "impact events"[33] and "anaesthesia related consequences"[34] from other studies of anaesthetic mishap. The studies were carried out in hospitals as far apart as Hong Kong,[28] Australia,[24 25 29] the United Kingdom,[23] North America,[26] and New Zealand,[27] many of which would probably have had quite different working practices. The most common events reported

113

and their associated factors are shown in boxes 4 and 5.

All the studies described induction and maintenance of anaesthesia as being the times when most problems arise, as opposed to emergence and recovery which were relatively free of untoward events. Only about half the studies, however, reported more mishaps associated with emergency cases, and two studies from the same department suggested there might be a slightly increased risk associated with paediatric cases.[24][25] It is alarming that two "critical incident" studies reported "teaching in progress" as a factor predisposing to adverse events.[1][29]

Contributions of Cooper's model

Many studies in which adaptations of Cooper's model of "criti-

---

Box 4 – Examples of the most commonly quoted "critical incidents"[1][18–20][22–29]

- Problems with the breathing circuit – disconnections, misconnections, and leaks
- Problems with giving drugs – overdose, underdose, and confusion of syringe or ampoule causing wrong drug to be given
- Problems with intubation and control of the airway – failed intubation, oesophageal intubation, endobronchial intubation, accidental or premature extubation, and aspiration
- Failure of equipment – problems with laryngoscopes, intravenous infusion devices, valves in the breathing circuit, and monitoring devices

---

Box 5 – Examples of the most commonly quoted "associated factors"[1][18–20][22–29]

- Inattention/carelessness
- Inexperience
- Haste
- Failure to check equipment
- Unfamiliarity with equipment
- Poor communication
- Restricted visual field
- Fatigue and decreased vigilance

---

cal incident" reporting were used have made contributions to knowledge about anaesthetic mishaps and potential mishaps. Research into the effect of the relief of one anaesthetist by another will be described followed by the special analysis of those "critical incidents" during which morbidity or mortality occurred. A large number of studies have related the capability of "critical incident" detection to the presence or absence of certain monitoring devices, and in some studies mock "critical incidents" have been set up in anaesthetic simulators.

Relief-associated incidents

In their first publication Cooper et al reported that nine of 359 preventable mishaps were associated with the relief of one anaesthetist by another.[1] In eight of the nine incidents it was the replacement anaesthetist who discovered either an incident or the cause of one. In only one case was the exchange of personnel regarded as a negative influence on the anaesthetic problem.

Later, Cooper et al attempted to analyse the features associated with various relief practices to design a safe and effective handover protocol. They examined their final database of 1089 "critical incidents" to investigate the effect of the relief process on the generation and resolution of the problems. There were 96 relief-associated "critical incidents" (incidents either caused or discovered by anaesthetists who had just assumed or were about to assume responsibility for the management of a patient). In most of these the relief process was thought to have had a beneficial effect in that the relieving anaesthetist was not responsible for initiating the "critical incident" but discovered either that there was a problem or the cause of a problem. Often direct communication with the departing anaesthetist, inspection of the circumstances, or examination of the anaesthetic record for trends in the vital signs or assessment of fluid balance, showed the impending predicament or its solution. Two conditions often detected by this process were hypovolaemia and endobronchial intubation. The mishaps which were caused by the relief process often resulted from poorly labelled syringes with unlabelled or mislabelled drug dilutions which resulted in a drug overdose or the wrong drug being given.

No morbidity or mortality was attributed to the relief-associated "critical incidents" in this study. Though fatigue was mentioned as an associated factor on only three occasions, the authors

115

suggested that it may have been present on other occasions and that there was a strong possibility that the relief of one anaesthetist by another (particularly during a long case) with a carefully constructed handover protocol may be beneficial. They stated that it would be difficult to provide more rigorous or more complete data on the effects of relief on the risk of anaesthesia. In addition, they postulated that the additional use of relief in the 244 mishaps not associated with relief in which fatigue, inattention, or boredom, were reported as contributing factors may have had a favourable effect.

In stark contrast to the beneficial effect of relief on anaesthetic risk described by Cooper et al, Currie, in a prospective survey of "critical events", reported 10 out of 167 citing the relief of one anaesthetist by another as an associated factor.[25] Although no specific details of the cases are given, *in nine out of the 10 it was considered to have precipitated the event.*

Substantive negative outcomes

Cooper et al examined the critical incidents which resulted in lasting harm to patients in great detail.[19] They defined a *substantive negative outcome* as mortality, cardiac arrest, cancelled operation, or extended stay in the recovery room, intensive care unit, or hospital. There were 70 cases including 25 deaths and 19 cardiac arrests in their database of 1089 "critical incidents." They wanted to discover whether any difference could be detected between these incidents and those which resulted in no harm at all. It was not clear why some errors produced injuries while others were detected and corrected promptly. They reported evidence of deficiencies in knowledge even in trained personnel which had contributed to some of the outcomes. This highlighted a need for in-service training about relatively new drugs, procedures, and equipment.

Though there were no more multiple critical incidents recorded with patients who had been injured in some way by an anaesthetic mishap, there were more "associated factors" reported with this subset of cases (3·4 associated factors/case compared with 2·5). The authors suggested that many adverse associated factors slowed recovery and reduced the margin for error. In addition the patients who were moderately or severely ill beforehand were more likely to come to harm if a critical incident occurred. Overall 41% of critical incident reports involved moderately or severely ill patients, but this figure increased to 71% of those with a "substantive negative outcome." They postulated that although the process of error was random, there is a smaller margin for error in sicker patients. This point was discussed by Gaba and is one aspect of what is described as tight coupling.[35] Galletly and Mushet suggested that several factors caused tight coupling in anaesthesia and hence a smaller margin for error – the use of neuromuscular blocking drugs, the presence of cardiorespiratory disease, certain types of operation, and the effect of the general anaesthetic agents in hastening physiological changes.[27] Looser coupling was produced by higher inspired oxygen, preoxygenation, and spontaneous breathing techniques.

There was also a difference in the proportion of equipment failures in the group of patients who suffered harm; 4·3% of the events with substantive negative outcomes involved equipment failure whereas this figure was 14% for the remainder. This suggested that there should be emphasis on the development of technological aids to vigilance and detection of error rather than on improving the reliability of equipment. Cooper et al said that one possible explanation for these results was that anaesthetists' own errors were more memorable than equipment failures, and that there could be a bias in the events that were remembered especially if they had an unhappy outcome.[19]

Relative usefulness of monitors

The direct failure of monitoring devices contributed to 6% of the database of frequently occurring incidents of Cooper's group.[20] In the same publication Newbower et al also suggested that besides these outright failures, lapses of the monitoring process occurred despite technically correct operation of the actual devices. Either the monitoring was ineffective in detecting the difficulty or the information displayed was not effectively absorbed by the anaesthetist. To examine this in more detail they assessed the efficacy of their current monitoring techniques in the prompt discovery of two types of difficulties: firstly, *patient disconnection* (as an example of a sudden event) and secondly, *hypovolaemia* (as an example of a gradual phenomenon).

Patient disconnection – Of 62 reported patient disconnections during mechanical ventilation (two of which resulted in death) the first things that were noticed that caused the discovery of the disconnection are shown in table I. Only half the discoveries were

117

TABLE I   Means of discovery of disconnections

	No of cases
Change in heart rate or blood pressure	16
Direct observation of the disconnected circuit (not necessarily at once)	15
The patient's colour	10
Changed performance of the ventilator	8
Absent breath sounds	8
Absent chest movements	7
Routine blood gas analysis	3
Changes on electrocardiogram	2
Cardiac arrest	1

Half the discoveries were made before there were any changes in the vital signs, and there were two deaths in the series.

made before any changes in the patient's signs. Besides initiating strong arguments for the adoption of low pressure alarms for every patient who is ventilated, this implied a lack of attention to various monitoring devices which must have been present – for example, the electrocardiogram and the oesophageal stethoscope. In five of the 62 incidents the disconnection was discovered by another anaesthetist who was relieving the primary anaesthetist for lunch or coffee. In three cases it was the abnormal result of routine blood gas analysis that prompted the discovery.

Hypovolaemia – There were 19 cases of hypovolaemia and almost all involved inexperience on the part of the anaesthetist. They were often discovered on exchange of personnel or review of vital signs by a more experienced anaesthetist. Technological sensors and instruments were not thought to be particularly important; lack of experience was blamed in some cases and lack of appreciation of the blood loss in others. The authors argued in favour of a more effective display of information such as trend plotting of vital signs and integrated effective alarm systems. They pointed out the obvious fallibility of human vigilance and advocated a search for the most cost-effective ways of increasing it.

Other critical incident studies

Other critical incident studies have been directed towards the relative usefulness of monitoring devices. Short *et al* in their departmental study found that capnometers were useful devices only when they displayed a continuous waveform.[28] In addition, they stressed the relative importance of backup systems to detect events when the primary monitor failed. They found the capnometer, the airway pressure monitor, and the spirometer were all theoretically able to detect leaks and disconnections in the breathing system but in practice each individual monitor failed sometimes so it was useful to have all three monitors. They also stated that the three most important monitors in the early detection of adverse events were pulse oximeter, end tidal carbon dioxide monitor, and airway pressure monitor.

Currie described 27 "monitor related events" in the analysis of 167 "critical events."[25] In six cases a faulty monitor or complication of an invasive monitoring technique contributed to the event described. In nine cases an available monitor was not used or was wrongly used. In three cases a monitor was not available which would have provided an early warning of a reported event. Finally, and most interestingly, on nine occasions a potentially lifethreatening event was detected early: by capnography (n = 5), by pulse oximeter (n = 2), by oxygen analyser (n = 1): and by oxygen failure warning (n − 1). McKay and Noble used the critical incident technique to investigate the usefulness of the pulse oximeter in the detection of adverse events.[32] They recorded a critical incident if "an unexpected physiologic change severe enough to require intervention by the anaesthetist to prevent a likely adverse outcome was signalled first by the oximeter." They concluded that the oximeter gave the earliest warning in at least 4% but maybe as many as 6% of cases. They presented a cost benefit analysis in favour of buying oximeters to prevent hypoxaemic episodes. It is important to note that electrocardiographic monitoring was probably used to corroborate the pulse oximeter reading in this study. When the oximeter alarm went off the recorded pulse rate was checked to see if it matched that of the patient. This would most probably have been done by the electrocardiographic trace as this was monitored routinely in all patients.

Newbower et al commented on the apparent ineffectiveness of electrocardiographic monitoring and in none of the studies using similar models of "critical incident" reporting is it listed among the useful monitors for detecting untoward events.[20] As they point out, however, part of the role of the electrocardiogram is to allow prompt detection of unexpected events such as arrhythmias or infarction. These may not be preventable or result from error and therefore would not be reported under Cooper's definition of a "critical incident." They also called for more sophisticated electrocardiographic monitors with arrhythmia alarms so they could aid vigilance without requiring constant observation.

The studies suggested that useful monitors should be identified; perhaps what is required is not more integrated monitors but fewer monitors more directly related to the patient's wellbeing.

Allnutt wrote about "the hope that a very real symbiosis between man and machine could allow each to counter the others weaknesses . . . the potential is there because man possesses attributes such as drive and intuition and pattern matching skills while machines are dispassionate, possess reliable and virtually unlimited memory and never tire of repetition."[21]

Simulated critical incidents

The efficacy of monitors in helping to avert anaesthetic disasters depends on how the information that is monitored and the clinical observations are used. Sometimes a problem is not perceived correctly because data contradictory to the original incorrect diagnosis are rejected. This may explain the positive effect of a change of personnel, when a fresh and often more experienced mind was helpful.[18] The method by which anaesthetists make decisions in the setting of dynamically changing information has been investigated using anaesthetic simulators. "Critical incidents" have been generated in the simulators and data about responses to them collected and analysed. Gaba and deAnda assessed the behaviour of anaesthetic trainees to these "critical incidents."[36] They found that circuit disconnection (which had figured prominently four years before as causing lasting morbidity and even mortality[19]) was routinely detected and corrected quickly. The monitors and alarms were highly effective in aiding even the inexperienced personnel to prevent negative outcomes. More subtle problems like endobronchial intubation and atrial fibrillation were more difficult to detect. Abnormal instrument readings were rejected as artefacts and subjects failed to use backup sources of data to check the readings. It was also found that multiple simultaneous audible alarms were confusing.

Unlike the almost life-like simulation of Gaba and deAnda, Schwid and O'Donnell produced a computer program that simulated many physiological and pharmacological aspects of general anaesthesia.[37] Ease of use, predicted patient responses, and suitability for training and evaluation of reactions to "critical incidents" were assessed in 44 residents and anaesthetists at seven training centres. The authors acknowledged that the program could not predict vigilance in the operating room, or manual skills, but after thorough familiarisation it could be used to assess cognitive skills. In subsequent work they assessed 30 anaesthesiologists (10 residents, 10 faculty anaesthesiologists, and 10 anaesthesiologists in private practice), on their management of six simulated cases which incorporated commonly reported "critical incidents."[38] These included oesophageal intubation, a cardiac arrest, and an anaphylactic reaction. Like Gaba and deAnda, Schwid and O'-Donnell described "fixation errors," when an initial faulty diagnosis was not reassessed in spite of conflicting clinical signs and deterioration of the patient. In addition, they reported that nine of 30 subjects tried to find the cause of a problem while undertreating severe hypotension.

The simulators were reported to be useful for determining patterns of management error for both experienced and inexperienced anaesthesiologists. They indicated that diagnostic and corrective protocols as well as vigilance were required for the successful management of adverse events. Berge *et al* reported the use of a simulator for detecting equipment failure in the anaesthetic machine.[39] They argued that several of the machine faults occurred so rarely that few anaesthetists would ever encounter them during their clinical practice. They pointed out that it is hazardous to make temporary defects in normal apparatus to facilitate teaching so they present the simulator as the optimal tool for showing such phenomena.

Simulators can be used to assess the ability of the anaesthetist to recognise diagnostic clues, make diagnoses rapidly, effect treatment, and evaluate a patient's response during their management.

Departmentally based studies

The value of the Cooper model of "critical incident" collection in an anaesthetic department can be illustrated by his first study from the anaesthetic department of one teaching hospital in Boston. Eight of 17 incidents of inadvertent low flow of oxygen were caused by the design of the control knob of the oxygen flow on the anaesthetic machine, which had been modified in the department so that it was easily distinguishable from the control knob of the nitrous oxide flow; the modification was the cause of the problem. In addition, numerous critical incident reports

121

described confusion with the common gas outlet on the anaesthetic machine and the scavenging port. As a result of these reports action was taken to prevent the problems. Cooper wrote "The square oxygen knob and the reservoir bag transposition incidents are examples of errors peculiar to institutional practices. They illustrate the need for evaluation before implementation. Procedures for controlling the kinds of equipment modification that might lead to incidents of this type are often informal at most institutions. Under present conditions many near misses and even serious accidents might occur before such situations were formally recognised and corrected."[1]

Craig and Wilson,[23] Kumar et al,[26] and Short et al[28] all described critical incident studies of this type as part of a departmental quality assurance programme. Currie et al ran a programme from a single department covering two teaching hospitals in Sydney and they described the "low level of inertia" of such studies allowing rapid evaluation, response, and feedback.[24]

Advantages and disadvantages of critical incident studies

The collection, analysis, and feedback of reports of adverse events and near misses in anaesthetic practice, resulting in the development of preventative strategies, is an essential part of any programme to promote quality and safety in anaesthesia.

Advantages

There are many advantages of Cooper's model of critical incident reporting. These include aspects of the actual study design, of the continuing nature of the studies and the ability to highlight the importance of apparently trivial events.

Study design – The study design that incorporates voluntary, anonymous reporting produces a high compliance rate and is probably essential for monitoring human error in particular. A bigger database is provided by the inclusion of potential as well as actual problems. The discussion of events focusing on prevention rather than blame creates a constructive atmosphere.

Assessment of preventive strategies – In a study with continuous reporting it is possible to identify problems as they happen and to see the effects of any preventive strategy. Similarly, the effect of buying a monitoring device and the evaluation of any other changes to equipment can be assessed before permanent changes are made.

Ability to highlight importance of apparently trivial events – Some seemingly trivial events have been highlighted as being important in the prevention of anaesthetic mishaps. For example, the mixing up of two syringes is a commonly reported event. There are virtually no case reports of this phenomenon so "critical incident reporting" has been the only means of highlighting its occurrence and working out methods (better labelling, discarding unlabelled syringes, and attention to having a place for everything on the worktop) to prevent it.

Disadvantages

Though they were of great value in their time, there are numerous disadvantages to the collection of "critical incident reports" as devised by Cooper *et al*. Some of these may have arisen because of the initial interest in the process of human error when the first studies were planned. There are problems with the definition of the data to be collected, with the terminology, and with the interpretation of the data. There are also problems of conflicting data and the limitation of human reporters.

Definitions – Many of the papers that have reported anaesthetic near misses have used slightly different names and definitions for the events collected (box 3). This has caused confusion about which events should be reported by participants, and may limit the comparability of data from different studies. It is therefore surprising how similar their findings are, though it probably means that the data are not specific. There is always the worry that the near misses are a different population of cases from the actual mishaps and collecting them together will confuse. Webb has described the absolute necessity for accurate data to aid in the cost benefit analysis for new equipment in the future.[40] In addition, if prospective trials of the effectiveness or otherwise of new monitoring equipment are to be carried out the data must be sound. This all argues for a firm, wide definition of the event to be collected with little confusion in the anaesthetist's mind (however inexperienced he is) as to what constitutes an event to be reported.

Terminology – From the first paper from Cooper's group about preventable anaesthetic mishaps,[1] it is evident that the term "critical incident" has been adopted from the technique as described by Flanagan.[9] The terminology has since become confusing. "An anaesthetic incident" in an Australian report is described as an event which does not necessarily have to include anaesthetic error or equipment failure and which may or may not be regarded as preventable.[41] In Canadian reports an "anaesthetic incident" has been portrayed as an adverse perioperative event with morbid consequences.[5] Gaba *et al* described how "through propagation and interaction," a simple incident may become a "critical incident" and "A critical incident which is associated with a substantive negative outcome may be considered an accident".[35] Galletly and Mushet defined a "critical state" as being when one or more system errors (defined in box 3) interact in some fashion and lead to an unstable condition from which a pathophysiological sequence begins to develop.[27] There is also an increasing tendency for anaesthetists to refer to any hazard as a critical incident.

For future studies the collection of "impact events"[33][42] or "anaesthesia related consequences"[34] (box 3) might be appropriate. The simplicity of collecting "real or potential adverse events" is as appealing as the definition is in the name. All terms have the advantage of preventing confusion with other phenomena in psychology or anaesthesia or the nuclear industry.

Misinterpretation of data – It should not be possible to extrapolate from critical incident studies to the actual percentages of mishaps that are the result of human error. One of the drawbacks of this type of work is the unknown amount of unreported data. Some of the authors of the prospective studies have tried to ascertain whether people are taking part in the studies by marking of cards[32] or by asking people in the study to indicate they had taken part.[23] It is still not possible to be sure and any quotation of the percentage of error or equipment failure emanating from such studies is suspect.

Conflicting data – The two studies that described adverse events in association with the relief of one anaesthetist by another were conflicting. Currie reported a negative effect from a prospective study[25] and Cooper *et al* reported a beneficial effect with data from interviews.[18] In view of the broadness of definitions, time scales, and working practices it is surprising there is not more conflicting data.

Limitations of human reporters – The limitations of human reporters particularly with a lapse in time since the reported event have been well described and are inescapable in this type of study.

The future

Studies of adverse events and near misses

Many anaesthetic departments already have critical incident reporting procedures that allow potential hazards to be identified and warnings to be issued immediately. In addition there are moves to provide national collection and coding of the incidents.[30][31][43] A new name and a broader definition of the events to be collected should be standardised and should not feature preventability, human error, or equipment failure. The aspects of anonymity and voluntary reporting should remain. Reports should be written on the same day so that there is the minimum of distortion and forms should be simple so that they can be filled in quickly.

Prospective studies by observers though expensive are probably the only effective method of discovering the true incidence of anaesthetic near misses and mishaps.

Directed studies

The effect of the relief of one anaesthetist by another should probably be re-examined in view of the conflicting data reported in the past.

The role of monitors could be studied from a new angle. The electrocardiogram monitor was rarely cited as helpful in the identification of adverse events, and there may be a danger that such monitors will be regarded as unnecessary particularly in times of financial strictures. It would be interesting to study the frequency with which a monitor provides some reassurance and help in theatre both in routine use and in difficult cases. It is possible that the electrocardiogram is the most useful monitor when the pulse oximeter fails as a result of artefact or hypotension.

Simulators

Simulators should be used to practise preventive strategies such as early action to identify, avert, and diagnose problems. It is possible that work in simulators may move towards assessing the behaviour of anaesthetists and identify those who are more likely to have accidents.

Gaba and deAnda described the detection of more subtle problems like hypovolaemia and endobronchial intubation as the next frontier.[36] This has been shown in both simulated and real critical incident reports to be more of a diagnostic problem for anaesthetists than a failure to detect one single lethal event such as oesophageal intubation or disconnection of the airway.

It might also be of interest to ask anaesthetists to fill in critical incident report forms after exposure to a set of standard critical incidents in a simulator to see how the accounts vary. The effect of the lapse of time on the accuracy of recall could also be evaluated by asking them to fill in the forms one week or one month later.

True critical incident technique

Cooper pointed out that "Although critical incidents are now often studied, the true critical incident method is not typically applied."[42] Sivarajan et al, however, used the critical incident technique to assess the performance of anaesthetists doing lumbar epidurals.[8] They indicated that the desired outcome of many therapeutic measures does not depend only on theoretical knowledge but also on the technical skills of physicians. While knowledge can be tested objectively in written examinations, technical skills cannot.

They set up the study to find out whether the performance of motor skills in the practice of epidural anaesthesia could be assessed reliably and objectively. They developed a list of 61 items in the form of a checklist under 11 categories. The categories included the performance of the technique, injection of the drug, and monitoring and assessing the level of blockade for up to 30 minutes. There were six items ("criterion" items) which required correct performance by the subject to pass the test. These consisted of the checking of resuscitation equipment and oxygen supply, the identification of the drug to be injected, and looking for blood and cerebrospinal fluid after inserting needles and catheters and aspirating catheters, and acting accordingly.

All but one of the eight subjects failed on one of the "criterion" items, usually failing to check the drug. They found that as well as evaluation of the performer, the skills test illuminated systematic errors in instruction which could be modified and improved. The study was elaborately prepared, and experts in the field of epidural anaesthesia defined the behaviour to be observed and measured. The details of their method should allow other centres to carry out similar work with far fewer resources.

There are many other areas of anaesthesia in which performance evaluation by a skills test would identify potential improvements in training techniques. Other aspects of the anaesthetist's behaviour could be studied in this way too, to see how often it falls short of the ideal. For the number of times the incorrect drug is actually given or an equipment failure is uncovered by an anaesthetic mishap, there must be numerous occasions when the correct drug was injected without being checked, or no equipment check was made but everything was in order. Research into the incidence of this sort of behaviour would be of great interest. Observers in theatre could record events as they happened with a check list of ideal behaviour.

The true critical incident technique could also be applied to such areas as optimal and inadequate categories of behaviour in an emergency, which might help to identify the ideal personality types to become anaesthetists. In a similar fashion perhaps research into anaesthetists who are prone to make mistakes or are more likely to have accidents would be rewarding.

1 Cooper JB, Newbower RS, Long CD, McPeek B. Preventable anesthesia mishaps: a study of human factors. *Anesthesiology* 1978;49:399–406.
2 Wallace-Barnhill GL, Florez G, Turndorf H, Craythorne WB. The effect of 24 hour duty on the performance of anesthesiology residents on vigilance, mood and memory tasks. *Anesthesiology* 1983;59:A460.
3 Norman J. Education in anaesthetic safety. *Br J Anaesth* 1987;59:922–7.
4 Lee RB. Why accidents happen. *Can J Anaesth* 1991;39:1030–1.
5 Armstrong JN, Davies JM. A systematic method for the investigation of anaesthetic incidents. *Can J Anaesth* 1991;38:1033–5.
6 Hardy JF, Taillefer J, Hébert Y. Critical incident report: total airway obstruction secondary to design of a tracheostomy set. *Can J Anaesth* 1991;38:936–7.
7 Gordon G. The development of a method of evaluating flying skill. *Personnel Psychology* 1950;3:71–84.
8 Sivarajan M, Lane PE, Miller EV, Liu P, Herr G, Willenkin R, *et al.* Performance evaluation: continuous lumbar epidural anesthesia skill test. *Anesth Analg* 1981;60: 543–7.
9 Flanagan JC. The critical incident technique. *Psychol Bull* 1954;51:327–58.
10 Andersson BE, Nilsson SG. Studies in the reliability and validity of the critical incident technique. *J Appl Physiol* 1964;48:398–403.
11 Wager CE, Sharon MI. Defining job requirements in terms of behaviour. *Personnel Administration* 1951;14:18–25.
12 Finkle RB. A study of the critical requirements of foremanship. *University of Pittsburgh Bulletin* 1950;46:291–7.
13 O'Donnell RJ. The development and evaluation of a test for predicting dental student performance. *University of Pittsburgh Bulletin* 1953;49:240–5.
14 Safren MA, Chapanis A. A critical incident study of hospital medication errors. *Hospitals* 1960;34:32–66.
15 Sanazaro PJ, Williamson JW. Physician performance and its effect on patients: a classification based on reports by internists, surgeons, pediatricians and obstetricians. *Med Care* 1970;8:299–308.
16 Waterston T. A critical incident study in child health. *Med Educ* 1988;22:27–31.
17 Blum LL. Equipment design and human limitations. *Anesthesiology* 1971;35:101–2.
18 Cooper JB, Long CD, Newbower RS, Philip JH. Critical incidents associated with intraoperative exchanges of anesthesia personnel. *Anesthesiology* 1982;56:456–61.
19 Cooper JB, Newbower RS, Kitz RJ. An analysis of major errors and equipment failures in anesthesia management: considerations for prevention and detection. *Anesthesiology* 1984;60:34–42.

20 Newbower RS, Cooper JB, Long CD. Failure analysis – the human element. In: Gravenstein JS, Newbower RS, Ream AK, Smith NT, eds. *Essential non-invasive monitoring in the operating room.* New York: Grune and Stratton, 1980:269–81.
21 Allnutt MF. Human factors in accidents. *Br J Anaesth* 1987;**59**:856–64.
22 Cooper JB, Newbower RS, Long CD. Human error in anesthesia management. In: Grundy BL, Gravenstein JS, eds. *Quality of care in anesthesia.* Springfield: Charles C Thomas, 1982:114–30.
23 Craig J, Wilson ME. A survey of anaesthetic misadventures. *Anaesthesia* 1981;**36**:933–6.
24 Currie M, Pybus DA, Torda TA. A prospective survey of anaesthetic critical events, a report on a pilot study of 88 cases. *Anaesth Intensive Care* 1988;**16**:103–7.
25 Currie M. A prospective survey of anaesthetic critical events in a teaching hospital. *Anaesth Intensive Care* 1989;**17**:403–11.
26 Kumar V, Barcellos WA, Mehta MP, Carter JG. An analysis of critical incidents in a teaching department for quality assurance. A survey of mishaps during anaesthesia. *Anaesthesia* 1988;**43**:879–83.
27 Galletly DC, Mushet NN. Anaesthesia system errors. *Anaesth Intensive Care* 1991;**19**:66–73.
28 Short TG, O'Regan A, Lew J, Oh TE. Critical incident reporting in an anaesthetic department quality assurance programme. *Anaesthesia* 1993;**48**:3–7.
29 Williamson JA, Webb RK, Pryor GL. Anaesthesia safety and the "critical incident" technique. *Australian Clinical Review* 1985;June:57–61.
30 Williamson J. Critical incident reporting in anaesthesia. *Anaesth Intensive Care* 1988;**16**:101–3.
31 Runciman WB. Report from the Australian Patient Safety Foundation: Australasian incident monitoring study. *Anaesth Intensive Care* 1989;**17**:107–8.
32 McKay WPS, Noble WH. Critical incidents detected by pulse oximetry during anaesthesia. *Can J Anaesth* 1988;**35**:265–9.
33 Cooper JB, Cullen DJ, Nemeskal R, Hoaglin DC, Gevirtz CC, Csete M, Venable C. Effects of information feedback and pulse oximetry on the incidence of anesthesia complications. *Anesthesiology* 1987;**67**:686–94.
34 Vaughan RW, Vaughan MS, Hagman RM, Cork RC. Predicting adverse outcomes during anesthesia and surgery by prospective risk assessment. *Anesthesiology* 1983;**59**:A132.
35 Gaba DM, Maxwell M, deAnda A. Anesthetic mishaps: breaking the chain of accident evolution. *Anesthesiology* 1987;**66**:670–6.
36 Gaba DM, deAnda A. The response of anesthesia trainees to simulated critical incidents. *Anesth Analg* 1989;**68**:444–51.
37 Schwid HA, O'Donnell D. The anesthesia simulator-recorder: a device to train and evaluate anesthesiologists' responses to critical incidents. *Anesthesiology* 1990;**72**:191–7.
38 Schwid HA, O'Donnell D. Anesthesiologists' management of simulated critical incidents. *Anesthesiology* 1992;**76**:495–501.
39 Berge JA, Gramstad L, Jensen O. A training simulator for detecting equipment failure in the anaesthetic machine. *Eur J Anaesthesiol* 1993;**10**:19–24.
40 Webb RK. Medical decision making and decision analysis. *Anaesth Intensive Care* 1988;**16**:107–9.
41 Morgan C. Incident reporting in anaesthesia. *Anaesth Intensive Care* 1988;**16**:98–100.
42 Cooper JB. How to measure what happens. *Can J Anaesth* 1991;**38**:1032–3.

8 Computers and medical audit

MICHAEL F FISHER

Computer hardware and systems are developing fast, so it would be inappropriate to try and produce a detailed assessment of the systems that are available now for medical audit, and anaesthetic audit in particular. I will therefore attempt to define the boundaries of the field in which the technology is to be applied and to discuss some of the important attributes that should be sought when specifying a computer system.

Firstly, however, it must be stated that a computer is not a prerequisite for medical audit. This is important, for just as no computer can compensate for a manager who cannot manage, a computer will be of no use for medical audit if the principles and methods of audit are not understood and applied. When diligently carried out, audit is expensive in terms of time and people. From it should stem a higher quality of patient care. Audit must be seen to work otherwise it is pointless, and the computer must play its part in making the whole process as cost effective as possible. Computers are relatively inexpensive, but the data gathering process is not, so decisions about what to audit and how to set about gathering the data to enter into the computer remain the essential tasks. It makes sense not to buy a computer system just to carry out "medical audit" if the computer can also earn its keep as a tool for the management and execution of everyday work. This will have positive cost benefit returns, and the data necessary for medical audit and quality assurance can be derived with little extra effort.

In this chapter I will describe a model for everyday anaesthetic audit, before suggesting a form of user and functional specification for a hypothetical computer system, and I will offer advice about buying a system.

129

Medical audit

The Report of the Standing Medical Advisory Committee defined medical audit as "the systematic, critical analysis of the quality of medical care, including the procedures used for diagnosis and treatment, the use of resources, and the resulting outcome and quality of life for the patient".[1] It went on to qualify this by stating that medical audit refers to the "assessment by peer review . . ." and that "The essential nature of medical audit is a frank discussion between doctors . . . without fear of criticism . . . on the quality of care provided as judged against standards. Confidentiality is essential." Box 1 shows the five elements necessary for effective medical audit.[2]

Box 1 – Five elements necessary for audit

- Peer review: an activity established and controlled by the profession
- Standards and quality: standards are set and monitored
- Patient based: this defines the need for confidentiality
- Systematic: a case conference alone is not enough
- Commitment to change in practice

Medical audit is based on both frank discussion by peers and confidentiality. From this a commitment to change is essential. For that discussion, the results of systematic analysis of clinical material must be available. Just collecting "figures" does not in itself constitute medical audit.

Clinical audit

The Standing Medical Advisory Committee Report makes a distinction between medical audit and clinical audit, the latter being described as involving an assessment of the totality of clinical activity and therefore having a multidisciplinary approach. Medical audit is a specialised subset of clinical audit. In either case it is the systematic analysis of clinical experience that provides the basis for the discussion and for which the computer may provide assistance.

Concurrent audit

This term was introduced by Rigby *et al* to describe the validation of processes or decisions as they are carried out.[2] For example, if the quality of record keeping is to be audited and certain standards set, and if a computer system is used to generate those records to that standard, then concurrent audit is being applied. In other fields this might mean the use of powerful expert and rule based systems to guide clinical activity. They see concurrent audit becoming increasingly prevalent as information systems develop in the health service.

Organisational audit

Donabedian suggested three components in the assessment of quality in health care: structure, process, and outcome.[3] Organisational audit is largely about the structure and processes within hospitals. The King's Fund has been responsible for initiating a form of nation-wide hospital audit called "organisational audit".[4] Hospitals volunteer not only to be audited, but also to provide assessors who visit other hospitals. Standards for this audit were initially set by the King's Fund but are themselves being modified in the light of experience. The audit is structured to encourage changes in the hospitals being assessed by having a two staged approach. First a comprehensive questionnaire is circulated, followed some months later by the visit of the team. The organisational audit of an anaesthetic department features in this scheme. Much of the King's Fund audit refers to structures within the department for which a computer is of little value. It is concerned with management design, accountability, and motivation of staff. It will also ensure that the necessary structure and processes for quality assurance have been set up, which will include the organisational aspects of anaesthetic care such as workload monitoring.

Anaesthetic audit

The Audit Committee of the College of Anaesthetists listed in its first report a number of desirable activities under the general heading of "anaesthetic audit"; these are shown in box 2.

The College recommendations are not, therefore, confined to medical or even clinical audit, and in terms of data acquisition they

131

Box 2 – Subjects to be covered by anaesthetic audit

- Logbooks for trainees
- Statistics of departmental service load
- Records of other departmental activities
- Morbidity and mortality
- Critical incident register
- Educational audit

---

represent a fairly wide range of activities. These are all either directly related to, or form part of the foundation for, the pursuit of quality in the service we provide to our patients, so it comes as no surprise to learn that the Audit Committee is now called the Quality of Practice Committee. Clinically, we should be concerned about the quality of the care we give to the patient in terms of both the technical quality of the anaesthetic and of the patient's recovery and memory of that anaesthetic. Organisationally, we should be concerned about the cost effectiveness of the service and the organisation of training within the department, because both of these will effect our ability to give anaesthetic care in the future.

Our overall aim therefore is quality of practice when all the facets of audit come together, and the specification of our computer system should reflect this. As it is the organisation rather than the computer that is the key factor in audit, consideration of two concepts from the United States may help in the design.

Medical management analysis (MMA)

Medical management analysis is a system of medical audit marketed as part of a quality assurance package for a total hospital environment. Like other audit systems in the United States it is not targeted at collecting data for resource management, but uses clinical records as a source of data for quality assurance. Coding of diagnosis and procedure is at the heart of the system, but MMA deals with "occurrence screening," which is a term used to describe "bad outcomes" and "inequality."

All records are screened by a team of "quality analysts" who evaluate records according to an objective list of criteria within 24 hours of admission and every 72 hours thereafter. If deviations are found action must be taken and the problem attributed and logged to one of four areas (box 3). If clinical judgment is involved the matter goes to peer review.

Of the 24 MMA criteria, 17 are relevant to anaesthetists (box 4). To put things in perspective, MMA is only one of 19 data sources used by a typical American hospital "quality assurance program" to identify problems or concerns in the organisation. Financial input is just one other. Most are clinically based. For a large hospital about 20 people of different grades are required to run this programme.

Box 3 – Possible sources of problems in occurrence screening

- Health care providers
- Hospital service departments
- Equipment
- Medical service

Box 4 – MMA criteria relevant to anaesthesia

- Admission as a result of poor outpatient management
- Readmission for complications or inadequate management on a previous occasion
- Irregularities in consent for operation
- Unplanned return to operation or delivery room
- Transfusion reactions or complications
- Hospital acquired infection
- Injury resulting from giving a drug
- Cardiac or respiratory arrest (low Apgar score)
- Unexpected transfer to special care unit
- "Other" complications
- Iatrogenic complication
- Falls and accidents; problems with infusions, drugs, or equipment
- Abnormal test results not investigated by physician
- Neurological deficit not present on admission
- Death
- Records not complete
- Dissatisfaction of patient or family

Quality assurance plan

Kuypers described a quality assurance plan for a small accident and emergency department (box 5).[6] He emphasises the value of using a computerised "log" to replace the extensive paperwork demanded by state and national bodies.

A model for anaesthetic audit: the user's requirement

Kuypers' model can form the basis for a good quality assurance plan in any hospital unit. Under this umbrella the requirements for an anaesthetic department might be as follows.

Policy and procedure committee

This committee consists of a core of medical staff (anaesthetists) who look at issues of medical audit in confidence, and a wider membership to consider clinical and organisational matters. It is concerned with the structure and processes within the department, reviews policy and sets standards against which the audit will measure outcome. Within this plan there will be need for a method of data acquisition that will form a foundation detailing the activity and output of the department from both a clinical and an organisational point of view. Small focused audits will also be required, which consider specific issues, obtain data, make recommendations, and review for evidence of change or compliance. This represents one of the greatest challenges for the computer as the software will have to be sufficiently flexible to cope with the different demands.

Box 5 – Aspects of quality assurance for a small accident and emergency department

- Review of policy and procedure
- Outcome monitoring
- Monitoring deviations from good patient care
- Risk management
- Patient complaints
- Incident reports
- Concerns of attending staff
- Review of continuing medical education

Statistics about the departmental service load are required to aid the departmental manager in securing adequate resources, and in using those that are already available to the greatest effect. Acquisition of these figures therefore ultimately becomes a quality issue and forms one of the baseline indicators in the quality assurance programme. As internal markets develop we expect to see incorporation of financial details as well. There is little choice here but to use computers if any degree of sophistication is required.

Outcome monitoring

Few departments of anaesthesia will have much routine data on outcome. The Society for Computing and Technology in Anaesthesia (SCATA) has championed the concept of a minimum data set for anaesthetic related data collection. Other than incidents or complications, including death, there is no reference to outcome. This reflects the difficulty of collecting such information in a large hospital and will be satisfactorily resolved only when hospital wide clinical information systems are in regular use. The interval between death and the most recent anaesthetic event should be stated. Other items that could reasonably match death as an outcome criterion are discharge intervals and reoperation rates (within a single hospital admission). We might also seek information on complication rates after anaesthesia, but these data are often difficult to define, let alone collect. For example, what is a "chest infection"? Somebody must make a diagnosis if the patient is to be treated correctly, but how is the computer going to know about it so that the event can be linked to an anaesthetic and form the basis of a medical audit report? The answer to this and other similar questions will be found as information technology develops in the NHS, and it represents one of the challenges for the next five years.

"Patient care occurrence monitoring"

"Patient care occurrence monitoring" has facets in all aspects of health care audit, as it looks for deviations from standards in patient care given. It is an expensive option if applied to the full as in medical management analysis, because many of the data required for the analysis come from scrutiny of the medical records. Nevertheless, given the advances in medical information technology that are now taking place we are likely to see development in this area. For example, we expect our anaesthetic information management system to be able to make associations to flag "occurrences" in the care of patients after anaesthetic which would indicate that further enquiries should be made as part of a focused audit study. Box 6 shows the "occurrence" *followed by a suggested data source.*

Risk management

All medical procedures carry risks. Risk management is a process of identifying the magnitude of those risks, categorising them in order of importance, and recommending protocols to reduce their incidence. Careful checking of patients in the anaesthetic room before operation is an example of risk management. Having identified that there is a risk of the wrong operation being done, procedures are put in place to minimise that risk. Of necessity the development of risk management protocols will depend upon the analysis of occurrence and outcome monitoring.

Box 6 – Patient care occurrence monitoring

Irregularities in consent to operation
- Mismatch between scheduled operation and operation actually carried out
- Operation cancelled due to inadequate consent

Unplanned return to operation/delivery room
- Unscheduled operation following scheduled procedure within the same admission episode

Transfusion reactions or complications
Cardiac or respiratory arrest
"Other" complications
- Intraoperative records
- Recovery records
- Pharmacy records
- Laboratory records

Accidents; problems with infusion, drugs, or equipment
- As critical incidents or complications

Death
- Patient administration system

Records not complete
- Presence of temporary records

Hospital acquired infection
- Antibiotic treatment during the postoperative period

Unexpected transfer to special care unit
- Patient administration system

Incident reports

Critical incidents are defined as occurrences during anaesthesia which if undetected will lead, or did lead, to a critical outcome for the patient. Cooper *et al* drew from the experience of "human factors" analysis of untoward events in the field of aviation.[7 8] Their two large studies of critical incidents were both conducted by interview and depended on the people concerned remembering the events. Looking to the future it would be better if the incidents were recorded as soon after their occurrence as possible. Here a computer could help. Analysis of such data is valuable in pinpointing potential hazards and in quantifying the response to educational or other corrective measures taken to reduce their likelihood. If no harm came to the patient, anonymity guarantees confidentiality and is thought to encourage full reporting. Incidents that harm the patient are complications and must be recorded as part of the clinical record. As in aviation, though, the strength of this technique depends not just on individual reports, but on the analysis of all reports from as wide a base as possible. Although Cooper *et al* described the use of a coding system for critical incidents, this seems to have been used only within their own study. A coding system is required which will allow critical incidents to be incorporated into a central database for analysis and reporting.

Continuing medical education review

Logbooks – The keeping of a logbook is a personal discipline and is most simply done with pen and paper using the College logbook format. Strang reported on the results of a questionnaire designed to find out how widely logbooks were used and noted that use declines with experience in the specialty and that even for frequent users less than half respondents claimed to have recorded all of their cases.[9] Those using computerised data collection featured the best. The advantage for the individual user comes when the computer is used to provide logbooks for staff with data generated in the everyday use of that computer in anaesthetic record keeping or theatre management.

Training reports – SCATA has proposed a standard form of training report and this has now been accepted by the Royal College (figure 1). The generation of such reports is a task ideally suited to a small departmental computer, but as always the real problem is acquiring the data.

St. SWITHUN'S ANAESTHETIC DEPARTMENT

TRAINING REPORT

From: 1.10.91   To: 30.3.92

FOR: Dr: J. Seaton   Grade: Registrar   No: 54

HOURS

	ELECTIVE	SCHEDULED	URGENT	EMERGENCY
Supervised:				
Unsupervised:				

	LISTED	UNLISTED
Supervised:	68	28
Unsupervised:	120	89
Supervision Rate:	36%	24%

CASES

SPECIALITY	TOTAL	SUPERVISED %	Gen	Ortho	Eye	Plastic	Other
Listed:	117	25	45	6	4	26	
Unlisted:	97	3	23	22		9	
TOTAL CASES	214	22	68	28	4	35	
< 6 months:	3	100	3				
Age: under 3 years:	8	100	3			5	
3–7 years:	13	54	5	2	1	3	
Over 80 years:	33	34	17	12	2	2	
Spinal blocks:	12	12	4	8			
Epidurals in theatre:	17	15	4	5		1	
Other regional blocks:	12	45		2		10	
Planned day cases:	23	13	7	1	4	17	

CAESAREAN SECTIONS

	Listed	Unlisted	GA:	Regional
Supervised:	9	17	13	13
Unsupervised:	18	7	12	13

ASA GRADE

ASA GRADE	1	2	3	4	5
Supervised:	44	10	5	2	1
Unsupervised:	97	40	15	0	0

(The above figures are for illustration only)

FIG 1—Sample training report (Society for Computing and Technology in Anaesthesia)

A brief functional specification

Overview

Two requirements seem to be important. Firstly, a wide range of data is required to create a foundation for quality assurance based on a series of quality indicators; these indicators will have to change and develop. Some of the information needed will be difficult to collect without a hospital wide clinical information system in place. Secondly, following on from the questions raised by the quality indicators, more conventional discrete audit studies will be undertaken. In both cases there has to be enormous flexibility in the design of the database and in the reporting techniques. Whatever the system, the user must be able to specify and design his own reports from the data available.

Whichever type of computer is chosen there will be a major problem caused by the large volumes of data that will be required at three discrete intervals (before, during, and after operation) and the means by which these data are handled will be important. Our goal was to find a computer that would be cost effective and would help the clinician in his everyday work. It is logical to make the core of the system the anaesthetic record.

Quite apart from the individual merits of automating anaesthetic record keeping, the rationale is that all the administrative audit data can be derived from the anaesthetic record, and the operative clinical audit can be simply dealt with. Yamamoto made a distinction between clinical and hospital administrative data in that the latter are categorised for statistical analysis, but as both types have to be collected and as administrative data are a subset of medical data, it makes sense to collect only the one and automatically convert to the other.[10] Data already collected as part of the preoperative assessment can be made available for the anaesthetist before induction and collated with laboratory information. Critical incident reporting can be included as part of the record, though retained in the system and not printed. If we include the recovery room in the net, this leaves postoperative outcome and occurrence reporting to be recorded, which will almost certainly depend on linkage to the hospital clinical information system or (as second best) input from routine discharge questionnaires at a later stage. The latter, however, will take time and effort to collect.

Ownership of data

Given that we need to collect sufficient volume and quality of data to enable the service to be assessed, and that the core data are collected by people going about their routine work, motivation of those responsible is important. The concept of ownership of the data being collected refers to the fact that each user of the system appreciates the personal relevance of those data and as a result has a vested interest in seeing that they are of the highest quality. It is inherent in this aim, therefore, that people will receive personal feedback about their activities and that the records collected are seen to be useful to their daily work.

Ownership of the system

A computer system is likely to be much more responsive to the needs of those using it if it is locally situated and controlled. The emphasis is on distributed processing using personal computers networked together. The local system is responsible for its own specialist data, but accesses the network for communally held data.

Security

Unauthorised access

A computer system based on clinical records and used for medical audit is likely to contain information that is sensitive both to patients and to the medical staff. As the information stored includes identifiable medical records, security measures must be taken to restrict access to those records. There must be controls to identify people who request access and to deny this as appropriate. Networked systems are obviously more at risk, but a locked office might be regarded as adequate security if the records are kept in one machine.

The Data Protection Act lays certain obligations on those who keep records on a computer where subjects can be identified. As far as medical audit is concerned, one way to avoid registration under the act is to depersonalise the records. Anonymity is recommended by the Standing Advisory Committee as a way of avoiding the risk of disclosure of information in legal cases. A good example of this is for critical incident reporting, but remember that members of staff are also "data subjects" if audit records contain identifiable references to them. The clinical records containing the details of individual complications are disclosable, but care has to be taken to guard the deliberations of the Policy and Procedures Committee and any subsequent peer review process from disclosure because this could be detrimental both to the staff and to the whole audit process. It follows that access to the computer on which the data are stored should be strictly limited and that generated audit reports should not be kept beyond their immediate period of relevance if they name individual people. It would be advantageous if the computer were programmed to depersonalise all audit reports automatically.

Tampering

There are many ways of using computer systems to gather data for medical audit and quality assurance purposes, and using a computer to collect and store identifiable medical records is one of them. If these records are to have any medicolegal credence then some assurance needs to be given that the records cannot be tampered with electronically once registered in the system, or perhaps, more importantly that if they are, then an audit trail must be left to show what changes were made, when and by whom. Optical disks are particularly suited for this purpose.

Backup

The Data Protection Act requires that measures are taken to prevent loss of data as well as to secure it from unauthorised access, so backing up must be routine. The optical disk can be duplicated or files can be transferred from hard disk on to magnetic tape systems. Larger systems will require power supplies that cannot be interrupted.

Software support

The user must have support when things go wrong and must be part of the security requirement of the system. The software should be underwritten by a reputable (usually commercial) organisation that is able to give that security.

Clinical audit

The practical problems of collecting background data for quality assurance fall into three obvious phases: before, during, and after the operation.

Preoperative audit

Anaesthetists today are faced with a number of problems result-

141

ing from changes in practice. One is the policy of admitting patients immediately before operation, which gives little opportunity for the traditional preoperative visit. Ideally, therefore, such patients should be seen by an anaesthetist in the outpatient clinic some time before operation, or fill in a preoperative screening questionnaire. Tompkin *et al* showed that a computer questionnaire may even be more accurate than a personal interview.[11] A properly constructed questionnaire can form part of a concurrent audit process whereby the audit itself becomes integral to the management of the patient. The computer system will therefore have to be capable of handling preoperative questionnaires. Whether these are entered on to a computer terminal or input in some other way (with an optical mark reader) it is possible to separate patients who *must* be seen by an anaesthetist (by implication in good time before the proposed operation) and those who need not be seen until shortly before anaesthesia. This questionnaire will form the basis of the operational system for preoperative assessment of patients. The answers to the questions must be available in the preoperative summary module of the anaesthetic chart before the patient arrives in theatre.

Operative audit

Operative audit of clinical anaesthesia is again concerned with quality. We are interested in the observance of policy decisions that have already been established and in avoiding complications and mishaps. Details of drugs are more appropriately associated with costing of anaesthesia and therefore form part of an administrative audit.

Record keeping – clinical audit should monitor the quality of the charting of the anaesthetic.

Complications arising as part of the anaesthetic are reported as clinical events. As part of the auditing process the departmental committee should review these cases.

Monitoring of patients is obviously a matter of current interest and the Association of Anaesthetists, through its guidelines on minimum monitoring, has effectively made this a significant item in any audit protocol.

Other points to be noted during the operation are shown in box 7.

Postoperative audit

Postoperative audit can deal with many issues, but provides the

---

Box 7 – Points to be audited during operation

- Timing of anaesthesia and operation
- Personnel taking part
- Categories of patients
- Type of anaesthetic
- Drugs or agents used

---

greatest challenge to our computer design. Examples of points to note are shown in box 8.

Problems of data collection

Techniques of data capture are the key to a good medical audit system. Data capture is expensive and it is not unusual for a hospital to employ several clerks specifically to enter medical audit data. It makes sense, therefore, to try and ensure that as much data entry as possible can be achieved as a by product of the routine work of the clinical staff. If the hospital has a network, then much of the routine data may be taken from the network (box 9).

Box 8 – Points to note in postoperative audit

- If the patient died and when
- That the patient recovered and the date of discharge
- How much postoperative analgesia was required
- Whether antiemetics were given
- Presence of fever (important for halothane and postoperative infection)
- Patient satisfaction (to include awareness under anaesthesia)

Box 9 – Data that may be taken from a network

- Patients' personal details
- Admission dates
- Laboratory results
- Data on death and discharge
- Operation and diagnostic codes

Ideally, if networking is available, no item of data should be stored twice. Typographical errors are common, and the only way to ensure a secure relationship between – for example, a hospital identification number and a patient's name – is for the association to be made only once. If separate computer systems in one hospital rely on separate entries of patients' personal information, then inevitably serious mistakes will occur.

The keyboard is still an efficient tool though it has been fashionable to ridicule it in favour of "graphical user interface" tools such as the mouse. The keyboard takes up space and is forbidding to the novice, but it is fixed spatially (a given key with its associated function is always in the same place) and it is generally reliable. Environmentally protected keyboards are available for wet or hazardous areas. With a keyboard it is possible for the experienced operator to anticipate the computer's request for data. Generally the keyboard will be used as part of a more sophisticated anaesthesia information management system. Miniature keyboards are used on pocket computers which are also used as data input terminals.

Bar codes are appealing because they are simple to use, and Ramayya reported a bar code system for anaesthetic audit.[12] They are good at picking up numerical data and are self checking, so as a means of entering patients' identification details they are second to none, provided that the bar code (in the form of a label) has been printed in advance. They have been used in a number of audit systems for many years, and menu books of codes are available for the user to scan, selecting those which are appropriate.

The drawbacks are the hardware used, and that they are not good for putting in random numerical or textual data because to do so a bar coded version of a keyboard would have to be created. A composite bar code and conventional keyboard would be required. The hardware must be first class with codes printed using the correct ink for the pick up wand in use. Some seemingly black inks are translucent to the red/infrared spectrum used.

The touch screen has instant appeal. The technology is fascinating to the novice and the screen design enables only relevant decision points of the program to be displayed. The disadvantage is that the user must see and identify the spatial position of those key points on the screen before action can be taken in contrast to the keyboard on which the keys are always in the same place. The use of the screen to replicate the keyboard to input text is a particular disadvantage.

The optical mark reader is a device that scans a page and detects pencil marks on the paper and relates them to a grid of expected returns, the importance of which is indicated by the design of the printed page and the location of the marks. This device is used for recording data for an anaesthetic audit.[13] Optical mark readers are highly suitable for "yes/no" answers and can return simple numerical data if the form is suitably designed. They are incapable of returning free text. They are used to collect simple audit data in anaesthesia – for example, "mark the box corresponding to the drug used for induction of anaesthesia." The paper record used to register these marks has in the past not been a complete record of an anaesthetic and therefore sometimes two records were required. This increases the work required of the anaesthetist. Recently, self carboned forms have been designed which offer an opportunity to combine optical mark reading and graphical charts with written text for inclusion in the patients' records. The techniques used for optical mark reading (the readers and the software used to drive them) must be chosen with care because the forms tend to be inflexible. They have to be reprinted if new drugs, techniques, or other particulars are introduced, and this means that the software used to drive the reading machine must be modified. Previously circulated forms must be removed from circulation or be self identifying in some way to avoid errors in the return of data which would otherwise be undetectable. User configurable and modifiable systems are available. Optical mark reading is of limited use for focused audit studies which require flexible reporting over short periods.

Portable computers

We have used portable computers for entering data since 1982,[14] and these have now been superseded by a full anaesthesia information management system. There are various types of portable computer in common use, but some of the small "pocket organiser" versions cannot be used to generate anaesthetic records but rather just gather records that are suitable only for workload and training records. This results in duplication of work which is best avoided. Portable computers have the advantage that they allow data to be entered at any anaesthetising location and are cheap.

Their disadvantages are that their software and displays are limited, and so they are not "user friendly." They invariably started as "in-house" systems and many have been developed into full commercial systems. Generally these computers have been pushed to their limits and cannot be upgraded as technology advances.

Personal computers

Ordinary personal computers have been used in operating theatres, but this cannot be advocated, simply as a matter of safety. Personal computers are not manufactured to the strict safety standards that apply to operating theatre equipment and should never be connected directly to patients. Tests have shown that some have large leakage currents, and there is also concern about hygiene and damage from spillage of conductive liquids and liquid volatile anaesthetic.

Digitising pads

Digitising pads are mentioned here for completeness. They have been around for many years but do not seem to have found a routine place in medical computing. The pad resembles a blotting pad which is constructed with a grid of sensors that can identify the location of an attached pen as X-Y co-ordinates. It is possible to superimpose paper forms on the pad and locate significant points with the pen to generate results similar to those of an optical mark reader. The pad can also recognise simple handwriting.

"Pen point" technology

The concepts of the touch screen and the digitising pad have now been incorporated into portable computers which use a pen to point at the screen. They are similar to a digitising pad but handwriting (block letters) can also be identified, and converted into a computer readable form for storage. These are attractive features, and it remains to be seen whether it will become popular. It is relatively expensive at present.

Graphic user interfaces

Programs that use graphic user interfaces have the attributes of a pleasing graphic screen design, standardised screen, and data

146

handling methods, and are therefore easier for the novice to manage. They use a pointing device (mouse or tracker ball) which, though it initially seems to be an advantage, has the same limitations as the touch screen. This is because the mouse is easiest to use with the operator sitting at a workstation. Much the same applies to the roller ball variant. Programs based on graphic user interfaces are much more complex to write than text based ones and are therefore going to be much more expensive for such a small market. The aim in the market is to produce generic products that can be easily modified by novice customers to suit their requirements. The new data handling products now go a long way towards solving the needs of database and report production. These programs have no advantage over the simpler text interface based ones as far as amounts of data that can be entered are concerned; input of data remains a key problem.

Automatic data uptake is in most cases a feature of only the most advanced anaesthesia record keeping systems, the data uptake mainly being from monitoring equipment attached to the patient. Links with hospital information systems should return up to date laboratory data and the patient's personal information.

Verification of data – If the computer system allows for entry of free text to important fields (usually when prearranged options are inadequate) then verification of data will be required at some point. This is expensive because it is time consuming and should be avoided if possible. All data for analysis should be coded.

Coding

As we are specifying a computer system for medical audit, storage and analysis will be required, and coding is essential. Firstly, it reduces storage space. It makes no sense to store the full name of a drug – say thiopentone sodium – in a record of an anaesthetic when we could just store the single character "T" which we have assigned as a code for the full name. Secondly, it makes subsequent processing much easier and faster because only one character has to be looked at to see that thiopentone was used. Thirdly, if "thiopentone" is put into the computer as free text every time, it is time consuming, and will lead to errors or abbreviations that the computer will be unable to recognise.

To use the code "T" for "thiopentone," although valid in its context, would be a bad example of coding because it is over simplistic and the coding system is limited in resolution to the number of upper and lower case letters in the alphabet. The codes used should be invisible to the user, but internal to the computer and allow the person entering the data to use natural language. This will, in most cases, involve selecting items from menus, but there are other options – for example, interaction between the screen and the keyboard in such a way that the choice narrows down to the required entry progressively with each key stroke. Coding may be intrinsic to a single computer or system, in which case codes will be meaningless to other systems. This is not necessarily a problem unless summarised records (codes) are needed for collation and reporting at a central location. Separate systems have the advantage that codes can be assigned automatically by the computer as new terms are required, but there can be no hierarchy of codes if they are randomly allocated. If more structure is required, or if individual records are to be transported between systems as codes, then an established coding system will have to be used.

In the past codes for diagnosis (International Classification of Diseases – ICD)[15] and surgical operations (Office of Population Censuses and Surveys – Classification of Surgical Operations Revision 4 – OPCS4)[16] were the principal ones required for central collation and all hospitals generated these codes for transmission to regional centres for Hospital Activity Analysis.

A general practitioner, Dr James Read, devised a simple set of four digit alphanumeric codes covering history and examination so that he could store his records on a computer and use the saved codes to generate letters and reports automatically. He then took the OPCS4 and ICD codes together with the British National Formulary and recoded them all to his standards. Together they formed the Read Clinical Classification. His work has now been recognised by the NHS Management Executive, and a National Centre for Coding and Classification has been established with Dr Read as its first director. The codes are now Crown copyright. The Centre is at present engaged on a massive and complex program to code the terms used in hospital medicine with a view to making them available in 1994 for use in *clinical* hospital (audit) systems. These aims are admirable and will greatly facilitate exchange of data between departmental systems. Anaesthetists are involved in defining the terms used in the specialty, and some hope that this will make the interchange of coded anaesthetic records feasible.

148

Specification of an anaesthetic audit computer system

Before buying a departmental computer it is worth looking at what is already available in the hospital.

Hospital information support system

A hospital information support system is unlikely to provide clinical information on a scale necessary to fulfil the total requirements for anaesthetic quality assurance, but it will contain much useful information that is otherwise hard to get such as details of deaths and discharges. Such systems are usually mainframes with a large (and expensive) central computer linked to scattered terminals. As a result it will be too inflexible to use as an audit system, and changes required for local needs will be virtually impossible. Generally the more distant the computer is from the site of the work, the less reliable and detailed the information becomes. Nevertheless, it should provide at least some information on outcome.

Operating theatre management systems

Ideally, the operating theatre management system should be a subsystem of the clinical system. Theatre managers who installed "stand alone" theatre management systems will appreciate the cost of entering data. Nevertheless, it will have been provided to give the theatre manager detailed figures on workload, much of which will be of value to the anaesthetic department. Some theatre management systems allow the incorporation of "audit" fields in their records, but this is unlikely to offer more than basic workload data and will be pretty inflexible. Data should be exported from the theatre management system into a suitable proprietary database for analysis and reporting.

Clinical hospital networks

Hospitals that had the foresight to install a computer network for clinicians to use with clear standards for communication offer the best chance for the development of medical audit. This leaves the local user with the responsibility for deciding how to implement a local system, but with a wealth of data available on line from the common pool of other users in other departments. Anaesthetists can then implement whichever system they wish, but obtain details of outcome and other data from the network.

Anaesthetic systems

It is not possible to give a specific recommendation for the purchase of a system, which will depend on local circumstances. Figure 2 shows the relation between the outlined audit objectives and the likely computer requirements in terms of gross scale. Three levels of computing requirements are proposed, though in reality the margins are blurred. The simplest is just a stand-alone microcomputer, moving up through a more dedicated system with semiautomated data capture, to the top of the range anaesthesia information management system. An anaesthesia information management system can be defined as a networked system with workstations at each anaesthetising site capable of generating full anaesthetic records, with appropriate means for data capture before and after operation and linked to a hospital information system.

For the simplest requirement (that of keeping personal logbooks and reporting critical incidents) a computer is of limited use, although a suitable program will be necessary if it is required to categorise and report centrally on critical incidents. If it is intended to make any use of the data stored in the logbooks, then data entry becomes an issue and the computer becomes more useful. The grey area shown in figure 2 is for focused small audit studies which may be conducted manually unless the data collection and management capability of the microcomputer is sufficiently flexible. If data entry is not a problem, then the latest

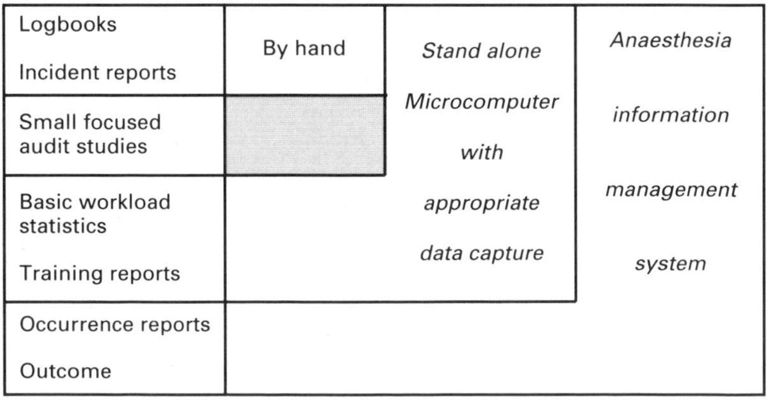

Logbooks Incident reports	By hand	*Stand alone*	*Anaesthesia*
Small focused audit studies		*Microcomputer* *with*	*information*
Basic workload statistics Training reports		*appropriate* *data capture*	*management* *system*
Occurrence reports Outcome			

FIG 2—Audit objectives and computer requirements

database management products on the market offer a good start. Some even offer the opportunity to extract data from other proprietary databases, so that switching between products is possible, but do not underestimate the time required to set up these programs, and particularly the time to enter the data required. There is a temptation to try and solve data handling requirements as "do it yourself" projects, but the work involved invariably exceeds the original estimates, the development is usually given to an "enthusiast" who leaves and takes the expertise with them, or the burden of data entry left to somebody in their spare time will prove too onerous.

To collect data about workload and for training reports a self contained microcomputer system will be adequate, as long as methods of collecting data are settled. Some form of semiautomated data collection is required even if you are working to the SCATA minimum data set. This involves the collection of at least 25 items on every patient and represents a serious amount of data handling. Semiautomated data entry techniques will be needed and this is generally not a task even for a dedicated enthusiast. Professional help will be required.

The practical choice at this simpler level is between optical mark reading forms, bar codes, and portable computers in the operating room. Cards may be completed at the time of anaesthesia and entered to computer centrally by keyboard, but it will be necessary to employ somebody to do this. Paper records can be kept that permit automated data entry (such as optical mark reading). Otherwise data will have to be entered directly on to the computer by bar code, keyboard, or semiautomatically and then transferred to the self contained computer for storage and analysis.

For a basic level of occurrence and outcome reporting, a full anaesthesia information management system is likely to be required if the costs of personnel needed to mount this kind of audit are to be contained. A full anaesthesia information management system should be specified with the capability for conducting small studies with appropriate means of data capture and reporting.

Outcome and occurrence reporting are likely to be the most rewarding of all the audit processes in terms of improvements in quality and efficiency. Through the use of such audit the anaesthetist might learn that induction drug A is not really of any benefit, or that postoperative bed days are reduced by the use of technique B. Furthermore, the organisational information derived from the clinical records will help managers and may save them money otherwise used to employ people to log paper forms through a "management computer system," or in finding ways of economising on drug bills. It is likely that only with a full anaesthesia information management system will the cost benefit analysis turn in favour of the computer system. The tools required to monitor these criteria will be expensive.

Purchasing considerations are well covered by Rigby *et al.*[2] As the issues of quality assurance transcend those of the rather more narrowly defined medical audit it is likely that those looking at information technology as a source of funding will do better than those who apply to medical audit budgets which seem to be poorly endowed.

In 1986 Gravenstein speculated on the likely use of computers in anaesthesia in the future.[17] While one might take issue with some of the clinical features in this article (such as servo controlled anaesthesia) most of the technical details have now, or are in the process of, being achieved.

Gremy urged us to keep in our minds, always, the single concept that lies behind all our work, that of *public health*.[18] Medical informatics is just one of the means by which we seek to help to promote, protect, and restore health.

1 Report of the Standing Medical Advisory Committee for the Secretaries of State for Health and Wales. *The quality of medical care.* London: HMSO, 1990.
2 Rigby M, McBride A, Shiels M. *Computers in medical audit.* London: Royal Society of Medicine, 1992.
3 Donabedian A. Evaluating the quality of medical care. *Milbank Memorial Fund Quarterly; Health and Society* 1966;**XLIV**:166–206.
4 Pitt C. The King's Fund organisational audit programme. *Network (Medical Audit)* 1991;4:8–10.
5 Audit Committee. *First report of the audit committee.* London: College of Anaesthetists of England, 1989.
6 Kuypers ME. Computerized log and integrated quality assessment program for the small emergency department. *QRB* 1989;144–50.
7 Cooper JB, Newbower RS, Long CD, McPeek B. Preventable anesthesia mishaps: a study of human factors. *Anesthesiology* 1978;**49**:399–406.
8 Cooper JB, Newbower RS, Kitz RJ. An analysis of major errors and equipment failures in anesthesia management: considerations for prevention and detection. *Anesthesiology* 1984;**60**:34–42.
9 Strang TI. Anaesthetic log books: are they being used? *Anaesthesia* 1993;**48**:69–74.
10 Yamamoto K. Design and use of medical record databases. *Med Inform* 1988;*13*:35–4.
11 Tompkins BM, Thompkins WJ, Loder E, Noonan AF. Computer assisted preanesthesia interview: value of a computer-generated summary of patient's historical information in the preanesthesia visit. *Anesth Analg* 1980;**59**:3–10.
12 Ramayya GP. AxAudit anaesthetic audit system. *Int J Clinic Monit Comput* 1992;**9**:149–58.
13 Verma R. A district wide anaesthetic audit. *Anaesthesia* 1991;**46**:143.

14 Fisher MF. Clinical experience of an in-house derived system for automated anaesthetic records. *Baillieres Clinical Anaesthesiology* 1990;**4**:47–65.
15 World Health Organisation. *International Classification of Diseases*. 9th ed. Geneva: WHO, 1978.
16 Offices of Population Censuses and Surveys. *Classification of surgical operations*. 4th rev. London: HMSO, 1987.
17 Gravenstein JS. Future use of computers in anaesthesia. *Int J Clinic Monit Comput* 1986;**3**:17–19.
18 Gremy F. Human meaning of medical informatics: reflections on its future and trends. *Med Inf* 1989;**14**:1–11.

9 Design of equipment for safety

R GREENBAUM

In the first half of the twentieth century many anaesthetists órdered custom-made machines to their own specifications. Nevertheless the Boyle machine evolved, and after 1917 pressure reducing valves (pressure regulators), rotameters, oxygen bypass, vaporisers, and a 22 mm conical fitting at the common gas outlet were incorporated. Governments found it necessary to design and build reliable machines with predictable performance during the second world war, and this allowed rational training of anaesthetists.

In 1955 a British Standard for medical gas cylinders was published which described the pin-index holes in cylinder valves and the corresponding mating pins on the yoke.[1] Only the correct gas cylinder attachment provides a pressure seal so that cylinder connections are gas-specific and not interchangeable among different gas services. This Standard applies to all gas cylinders up to a capacity of 4·5 l and also describes the colour code and labelling requirements for all medical gas cylinders. These requirements are incorporated in the International Standard ISO/R407[2] and the colour code in ISO/32.[3]

Unfortunately Germany and the United States did not adopt the international colour identification, and continue to indicate oxygen with blue in Germany and green in the United States. It is likely, however, that the ISO/32 colours will be adopted throughout Europe in the near future.

Modern anaesthetic machines include many other design features to minimise the risk of giving incorrect or hypoxic gas mixtures, to achieve satisfactory performance and accuracy of all

154

controls, and to facilitate interchangeability among apparatus made by different manufacturers. British Standard BS 4272, 1989,[4] specified the performance of continuous flow anaesthetic machines but specifically excluded machines that incorporated electrical devices. Other countries have either adopted the International Standard ISO 5358,[5] which was first published in 1980 and reissued in 1992, or like the United Kingdom, United States, and Australia have adopted many of the clauses of ISO 5358 as the basis for their own national standard. The end of the era of cyclopropane, ethylene, and ether anaesthesia has led to removal of designs suitable for use with inflammable and explosive agents and the need for antistatic specifications.

The rapid improvement in the availability and reliability of electronic and microprocessor controls and monitors has led to the concept of electronic surveillance of the anaesthetic work area proposed by Schreiber and Schreiber.[6]

Electronic surveillance accepts the monitoring recommendations of such bodies as the Association of Anaesthetists of Great Britain and Ireland[7] and the similar recommendations of other national professional associations. It proposes that the monitors and their associated alarms are integrated with the anaesthetic machine, ventilator, and breathing system to form an "anaesthetic work station." A *Draft standard for anaesthetic work stations* and their modes has been produced by the European Committee for Standardisation, and the configuration proposed in this draft document for protection of the patient against hazardous output is shown in table I. The committee may review or reject this table when the standard is published.

Many manufacturers believe that safety can only be achieved when a fully integrated system is supplied complete by one manufacturer, who is then responsible for all the equipment from the pipeline inlet via the patient to the anaesthetic gas scavenging system. Modular systems are being manufactured and it may be possible to integrate their alarm and monitoring functions to simplify the user checks so that they are comparable to a totally integrated work station.

The results of recent surveys have suggested that the mortality resulting primarily from anaesthesia has fallen to much less than 1 in 10 000 reported in 1982 (see chapter 7).[8] Most failures are the result of human error and probably less than 10% of anaesthetic accidents are caused by faulty equipment. Many of the "human

155

TABLE I   Anaesthetic work station configuration for protection against hazardous output

Actuator modules	Power failure alarm	Oxygen supply failure alarm	Inspired oxygen concentration		Anaesthetic agent concentration			Airway pressure			Exhaled volume		Breath system integration	Carbon dioxide concentration			Cut off device	AGSS	Maximal pressure limitation	Adjustable pressure limitation
			M	L	M	H	L	M	H	L	M	L		M	H	L				
Driving power																				
Electric	+																			
Pneumatic	+																			
Gas delivery																				
Oxygen		+	+	●																
Air			+	+																
Half oxygen and half nitrous oxide			+	+															+		
Others			+	+													+	+		
Anaesthetic vapour delivery module					+	+													+		
Anaesthetic ventilator module					+			●	+	+	●	+	+	+	+					+	+
Anaesthetic breathing system					●			●			●		●	+	+	+				+	●

Conditional requirement. M = Measurement; H = high level alarm; L = low level alarm. + = required; « = optional.

errors," however, do involve failure to use the equipment properly, to use the monitors and alarms, and to develop appropriate algorithms in response to changes in variables being monitored. Well designed machines can prevent or at least ameliorate the effects of an error, whereas poorly designed equipment is often cited as the cause of an accident. Allnutt stated that what a pilot in an aircraft (or a doctor) requires from his instruments is clear, concise, reliable, unambiguous, information to the accuracy (but no more) that he needs; and the controls must be comfortable, precise, easy to operate, unambiguous, and give him immediate and adequate feedback that his intended action has been effected. Displays and controls must be easy to use, and grouped logically by function and information flow.[9]

Current standards include visibility and ergonomic design requirements and urge the rational use of alarm signals.

Engineering concepts in the safety of medical equipment

The electrical and safety requirements of the International Electrotechnical Commission (IEC) 606-1 (identical to BS5724) apply to most machines, ventilators, and monitors used in anaesthesia and intensive care.[10] In certain cases particular standards have been written based on IEC 606-1 (the general standard), which take precedence over the requirements of the general standard.

IEC 601-1 is a large and complex document that includes requirements for stability, transportability, protection against mechanical hazards from unwanted or excessive radiation, explosions, excessive temperatures, and electric shocks. As most modern equipment has electronic components, current European (CEN) and International Standards (ISO) are being written in the format of IEC 601-1. Particular standards include anaesthetic gas monitors, capnometers, anaesthetic work stations, oxygen analysers, lung ventilators, and automatic cycling blood pressure monitoring equipment.

Equipment in which a single means for protection against a safety hazard is defective or a single abnormal condition is present is designated single fault condition. IEC 601-1 requires equipment to be safe, in normal use, or in single fault condition. Specific examples of single faults are shown in box 1. The implication of

157

Box 1 – Examples of "single faults"

- Interruption of protective earth conductor
- Interruption of one supply conductor
- Appearance of external voltage on floating applied part of equipment, signal input, or signal output
- Failure of electrical, mechanical, or temperature limiting component that might cause a safety hazard

---

these single fault requirements is that back up safety features must be designed into equipment so that the essential safety of the equipment is not lost when one component fails.

In automobile engineering, active safety devices that help avoid accidents include ABS braking or power assisted braking, whereas passive safety devices that protect the user after an accident include seat belts or air bags. In medical equipment pin-index safety systems for medical gas cylinders or non-interchangeable screw threads for medical gas pipelines are active devices whereas the nitrous oxide cut-off is a passive device.

In European standards, both the patient and operator must be protected against hazards from the delivery of energy or substances. Any device which can supply energy such as pressure or electricity or substances such as anaesthetic agents or hypoxic atmospheres are designated "actuators." Ways in which patients may be protected are shown in box 2.

The second and third modules require active intervention by the operator. This concept is illustrated by the actuator modules, protection, alarm, and monitoring modules proposed for the European standard on anaesthetic work stations (table I).

Box 2 – Modules that protect patients

- A protection module without the intervention of the operator protects the patient against hazardous output from incorrect delivery of energy or substances
- An "alarm module" provides a visual or auditory signal, or both, when an alarm condition is present
- A monitoring module displays or indicates a variable

Alarms

Many manufacturers and government departments in some developed countries want to see all compulsory monitors and all power sources supplied with both auditory and visual alarms. Schreiber and Schreiber stated that "the most important attribute of the anaesthetic monitoring system is a uniform and structured alarm strategy."[6] This strategy is aimed towards reducing the confusion caused by the increasing proliferation of alarm signals in the operating theatre while minimising the time required to recognise a problem and activate the alarm system. The classification proposed by Schreiber and Schreiber has been adapted in the Draft ISO 9703 and is shown in Table II.[6] They also proposed a system-wide alarm priority structure, the suppression of lower priority alarm signals, a centralised alarm display screen, and a single system-wide (temporary) audio silence button. Many alarms are outside the scope of the anaesthetic work station or ventilator, however, including syringe drivers, surgical diathermy, and laser, and so the proliferation of complex auditory alarms is, in my view, to be deprecated.

The problems of locating the source of a sound have been met by the use of harmonics to which the human ear is sensitive. These proposed signals are complicated, and this is illustrated by this quotation from the introduction to the current CEN draft on auditory alarms.

TABLE II   Alarm priorities and characteristics of signals

Alarm category	Operator response	Meaning	Indicator colour	Flashing frequency
High priority	Immediate response to deal with a hazardous situation	Emergency	Red	1·4–0·8 Hz
Medium priority	Prompt response to a hazardous situation	Abnormal	Yellow	0·4–0·8 Hz
Low priority	Awareness	Change of status	Yellow	Constant

"The auditory signals specified in the draft are somewhat akin to atonal melodies with specific temporal patterns, pitch patterns and timbres. Construction of the signal falls into two distinct phases, the specification of a pulse of sound which determines the timbre of the signal, and the specification of a burst of sound. The burst is produced by playing the pulse several times, at different pitches, with variable time intervals between them and at different amplitudes. The specification of the pulse involves specifying the spectral components of the signal and the specification of the burst involves specifying the temporal and melodic parameters."

Objections to the proposals were summarised by Sugg (box 3).[11]

The advances in technology in the 1990s should allow auditory signals to be used only to catch the attention of the staff. All information on the urgency and cause of the alarm can be displayed on screens or panels, so reducing the reliance on auditory signals and emphasising the role of visual displays. This line of development should reduce the number of spurious alarms, which is reported to be three quarters of all alarms during anaesthesia. Only 31% of alarms indicate a risk to the patient.[12]

Choosing the setting of alarm limits creates further problems, as the user may wish to change the limits. For example, during the course of an anaesthetic, the anaesthetist may want a high limit of volatile agent percentage during the induction, which is lowered as uptake of the anaesthetic proceeds. During recovery no low limit alarm is necessary. The user does not want to find a monitor with alarm limits set by the previous user – and so the alarm limits must automatically reset to the manufacturer's clearly visible predetermined default values. Few alarms satisfy these requirements.

Visual alarms are less contentious as they produce less disturb-

---

Box 3 – Objections to the CEN draft on auditory alarms

- The 12 specific risk sounds and grades of urgency are too complex to be remembered by hospital staff
- The analogy between a flight deck and intensive care or theatre environment is hugely misleading
- The cost is disproportionately high
- The concept is too detailed and design restrictive
- No clinical trials have been undertaken

ance and are compatible with IEC 601-1. A draft specification for visual alarm signals for anaesthesia and respiratory care has been issued for public comment. The main hazards to the patient arising from anaesthetic equipment are shown in box 4.

Design features to prevent hypoxia

Prevention of hypoxic gas mixtures reaching the machine:
- All medical gas cylinder inlet connections to anaesthetic machines (hangar yokes) shall have pin-index safety systems complying with ISO 407.
- Pipeline inlet connections for medical gases shall use the body of a non-interchangeable screw thread to connect, complying with ISO 5359.[13] In the United States a non-metric diameter index safety system is used.

These features have drastically reduced the number of accidents compared with the 1950s.

Prevention of hypoxic gas mixtures occurring at the machine:
- Always have the capacity for one oxygen cylinder, even on machines designed for use with a pipeline.
- Newer standards require that a method of interruption shall be incorporated in the gas flow control system to prevent the delivery of gas mixtures with oxygen concentrations of less than 21% in the fresh gas. This can be achieved by a mechanical linkage between oxygen and nitrous oxide flow controls. Alternatively, the differential pressure between the oxygen and nitrous oxide can be detected and the nitrous oxide flow controlled to maintain a safe percentage of oxygen. Machines may also provide a basal flow of oxygen at all times. There have, however, been reports of potentially lethal malfunctions of such systems.[14] These devices do not protect

---

Box 4 – Main hazards to patients of anaesthetic equipment

- Hypoxia
- Hypoventilation or hyperventilation
- Barotrauma

- Overdose or underdose of volatile anaesthetic
- Burns
- Electrocution

---

against hypoxia if a third oxygen free gas (other than nitrous oxide) is used.

- Few countries use carbon dioxide in their anaesthetic machines, but where carbon dioxide flowmeters are provided, hypercarbia and hypoxia have been reported as a result of inadvertently giving large flows of carbon dioxide. BS 4272 has been amended to state that when the carbon dioxide flow control valve is fully open, the delivered carbon dioxide flow shall not exceed 0·6 l/minute and, at this flow, the bobbin or ball float shall be in the lower three quarters of the visible section of the flowmeter tube.[4]
- ISO 5358 requires flowmeters to be accurate within 10% of the indicated value, between 10% of full scale, or 300 ml/minute, whichever is the greater.[15] In BS 4272 the required 10% of the indicated value has to be achieved at all flowmeter graduations.[4]
- There is widespread use of gas blenders which produce mixtures of oxygen with other medical gases, the proportions and flows of which are controllable and which prevent the production of hypoxic mixtures. There have been occurrences of backflow into medical gas pipelines and other hazards.[16]
- A gas cut-off device senses a fall in oxygen concentration or pressure and either cuts off the flow of nitrous oxide to the common gas outlet or reduces the flow of other gases to maintain a preset proportion of oxygen until the oxygen supply finally fails. The nitrous oxide is then cut off. The gas cut-off device is activated only after the oxygen supply failure alarm is activated.
- Oxygen supply failure alarm – there should be an auditory (with or without visual) alarm signal to indicate a fall in oxygen supply (whether pipeline or cylinder). If it is electrically powered it must be a high priority (immediate response) alarm.
- Oxygen analysers should be used to monitor fresh gas oxygen concentration close to the common gas outlet. Schreiber reported that an oxygen analyser was the single most important measure in the prevention of hypoxia, and analysers are compulsory in Germany and the United States.[17]

An oxygen analyser at the common gas outlet will detect that the wrong gas has been supplied at the oxygen pipeline or cylinder inlet; reduction or cessation of the pipeline or cylinder supply (unless 100% oxygen is being administered); incorrect flow control settings, and errors in flowmeters. An oxygen analyser in this position with an associated alarm will give the operator early warning of one of these events.

Hypoxia may also be produced by leakage of fresh gas at vaporiser connections, from failure to connect fresh gas to a circle breathing system or inadequate fresh gas supply into a breathing system, or disconnection within a breathing system (for example, the inner tube of a Bain system). It is therefore advantageous to monitor oxygen concentration in the inspiratory limb of a circle breathing system or at the patient connection port. If the oxygen concentration is to be monitored in one position only, the breathing system location is therefore preferable. In the anaesthetic machine check list suggested by the Association of Anaesthetists, the oxygen concentration should be measured at the common gas outlet.[18]

The development of fast response paramagnetic oxygen analysers has made breath-by-breath oxygen analysis more readily available than when mass spectrometers were required. An increasing difference between inspiratory and end-tidal oxygen concentration is a sensitive indicator of hypoventilation and precedes changes in oxygen saturation.[19] The "oxygram" sensor should be sited at the patient connection port.

Oxygen analysers are only just reaching acceptable reliability. In a recent review of the use of the checklist on 50 anaesthetic machines, 13 oxygen analysers were missing from machines – 12 away for repair and one defective.[20] It was noted that of their stock of 55 oxygen analysers, only 33 were present and in full working order. In my own hospital, a modern anaesthetic machine has an integral oxygen analyser that automatically cuts off the flow of nitrous oxide if it "sees" less than 25% oxygen. A fault in the analyser has made the machine unusable on several occasions.

Overventilation or underventilation

Accidents to patients caused by underventilation are still reported. The proposed European CEN standard recommends that airway pressure should be monitored, and that all breathing systems should include a means of monitoring end-tidal carbon dioxide.

When a ventilator is used in anaesthesia, both pressure monitoring and capnography are likely to be compulsory. Measurement of expiratory tidal or minute volume is compulsory for all ventilators with the exception of those intended for neonates (Table I).

163

*Breathing system integrity (disconnection) and breathing system
leakage*

Anaesthetic machines and ventilators that comply with international standards have 15 mm or 22 mm conical connectors made
to the precise and testable dimensional requirements of ISO 5356
Part I.[21] If these connectors are put together with a push-twist
action they give a good secure fit. Unfortunately, many cheaper
plastic components have now been marketed that do not satisfy the
gauging test of ISO 5356 Part I and produce insecure connections.

Part II of ISO 5356 gives specifications for screw-threaded
weight bearing connectors. These female components are compatible with the 22 mm male conical connector of Part I of the
standard and are intended for use at the common gas outlet of
anaesthetic machines or a ventilator port at which heavy accessor-
ies may be mounted.[22]

Repeated reports of accidental disconnection of breathing systems have, however, led to the development of a standard for a
latching connector – a female 22 mm fitting which incorporates a
latching mechanism. Latching connectors are required to maintain
secure engagement with a male 22 mm conical fitting when tested
at 37°C and at least 80% humidity with an axial separation force of
50 N and a torque of 25 N/cm. Unfortunately latching connectors
are currently being developed only for 22 mm connectors, yet the
commonest site of disconnection is at the tracheal tube 15 mm
connector. There has been strong resistance from some anaesthetists to a secure 15 mm connection. They believe that 15 mm
connectors act as a "fuse" or "weak link" which prevents accidental extubation of the patient should the breathing system be
inadvertently tugged, but tracheal tube connectors have never
been designed with this safety action in mind.

The other prime site for disconnection is at the common gas
outlet. After disconnection at this site there is no fresh gas flow; if a
circle absorption system or Bain system is used with a ventilator,
there will be some decrease in tidal volume and peak airway
pressure, but the ventilator will still produce an increase in airway
pressure and may satisfy a pressure operated ventilator disconnect
alarm and an oxygen analyser at the common gas outlet.[23] In the
United States, manufacturer specific locking devices are in widespread use at this site. The other common cause of leakage of gas
before the common gas outlet is faulty connections of user-
detachable vaporisers.

Indications of leakage may be shown by changes in the expired tidal and minute volumes, and the end-expired carbon dioxide and breathing system oxygen analysers. Ventilators of the type which has a descending movement of its bellows during exhalation will continue to move normally even after total disconnection, so ascending bellows ventilators are preferable.

Disconnect alarms are in widespread use. The most common mechanism is by pressure activation, and the pressure may be user adjustable. Disconnect alarms or apnoea alarms may also be activated by the expired volume or capnometer. It is essential to test the efficacy of a disconnect alarm by sequential disconnection at all possible sites.

Barotrauma

High pressure gas from cylinders or hospital medical gas pipelines has to reach the patient at respiratory pressures. Machines in the United Kingdom receive pipeline gas at 400 kPa and regulate cylinder pressure to this level. Many machines reduce the pressure further before it reaches the flow control valves.

The pressure at the common gas outlet is required to be between 35 kPa and 80 kPa so that occlusion at the common gas outlet will not damage the vaporisers and flowmeters (and so injure the operator and the patient). This relatively high pressure is required if fresh gas is to power the "minute volume divider" type of ventilators.

It is proposed that anaesthetic breathing systems and ventilators should incorporate a means to limit pressure to not more than 8 kPa (80 cm of water) (unless a special user-adjustable valve plus a fixed pressure limit of 12·5 kPa (125 cm of water) is requested). Reservoir bags complying with ISO 5362 have a compliance which limits pressure to 50–70 cm of water. The proposed European standard requires airway pressure to be monitored in the breathing system. Ventilator pressure monitors should also incorporate high pressure and low pressure alarms.

Barotrauma is still possible despite these safety measures when a single fault develops in the system. Perhaps the most common cause is user misconnection of a circle breathing system so that the reservoir bag port is confused with the expiratory port. In the United Kingdom the reservoir bag port has typically been vertical whereas the inspiratory and expiratory ports were horizontal. The new international standard ISO 8835, however, allows the reservoir bag post to be within 20° of vertical and the inspiratory and expiratory ports to be within 50° of horizontal.[25] As these three ports are all male – designed to accept a breathing tube pushed over them – mistakes are easy to make. Only careful reading of the marking and checking the system before use therefore will prevent accidents.

Overdose or underdose of anaesthetic agent

In some countries, the requirements for monitoring make the use of an analyser compulsory for the volatile anaesthetic agent, to check the performance of the vaporiser. If the alarm limits are set appropriately it should prevent overdose of the volatile agent because of a faulty or incorrectly set vaporiser. The appropriate site for a vaporiser-safety monitor would be immediately downstream of the vaporiser, but recent vaporisers are highly reliable and conform to the International Standard 5358 which gives detailed tests for the affects of high gas flow, back pressure, and over-filling.[15] It is therefore more usual and acceptable to monitor the vapour concentration in the breathing system as this will differ from the vaporiser output during anaesthesia with low-flow circle breathing systems.

The low concentration alarm is designed to alert the anaesthetist before the patient becomes "aware" as a result of an inadvertently low vaporiser setting (or an empty vaporiser). Unfortunately, these alarm settings require repeated adjustment by the user as widely different vapour concentrations are required during induction, maintenance, and recovery from anaesthesia.

To prevent inadvertent filling of vaporisers with the incorrect agent, agent-specific vaporiser filling systems have been developed. These were quickly accepted in the national standards of Canada and Germany, but some countries were worried by the lack of control of the bottle and bottle-neck sizes. Manufacturers of vaporiser and filling adaptors could specify one end of the system and could provide agent-specific bottle collars, but it is still possible to fit a bottle of a well known antiseptic to the bottle filling adaptor. Nevertheless, agent-specific filling systems are now widely supported and likely to be adopted throughout Europe. The final responsibility rests with the user who must read the labels of all drugs, including volatile anaesthetic agents.

Burns and fires

The general protective clauses given in IEC 601-1 (the general standard), section seven, describe protection of all medical equipment against excessive temperatures, fires, and other safety hazards.[10] Equipment which is designed to work at high temperatures such as humidifiers has specific safety requirements written for the special hazard associated with its use.

The general standard describes the maximum temperature of accessible surfaces of handles or knobs which are continuously held by the operator in normal use (55°C if metal) or held for short periods – for example, switches (60°C if metal). Any part of the equipment which may, in normal use, have a brief contact with a patient should not have a temperature exceeding 50°C, but otherwise it should not exceed 41°C. It is noteworthy that the use of antistatic or electrically conductive tubes is not recommended as high frequency surgical equipment may cause burns to the patient if the diathermy is close to the conductive tube.

If explosive agents were to be used, conductive tubes would of course be essential, but inflammable or explosive agents are being withdrawn and few developed countries allow their use. Though halothane will form flammable mixtures with oxygen and nitrous oxide when tested with high ignition energy there have been no reports of any injuries caused by ignition of halothane and so it is not necessary to have the APG safety features required for ether and cyclopropane on equipment designed to be used with halothane, enflurane, isoflurane, sevoflurane, or desflurane.

Materials which will not burn in air will ignite in oxygen or nitrous oxide, so electrical components which might ignite in oxygen or nitrous oxide enriched atmospheres must have a barrier between them and the oxygen, or have a ventilation system.

Any electrical circuit that can produce sparks or generate increased surface temperature must not have a surface temperature exceeding 300°C and an electrical-power rated as a no load voltage and short circuit current not exceeding 10 VA. External exhaust outlets should also be located at least 25 cm from any potential source of electrical sparks.

Electrical safety

The general safety requirements of IEC 601-1 describe all aspects of electrical safety in great technical detail. All electrically

167

powered equipment to be used on patients must be tested before it is used on patients and must satisfy the many requirements of this standard. This task is specialised and normally performed by trained medical physicists or engineers. The tests include measurement of electrical isolation from mains voltage.

Emergency equipment such as defibrillators, and routine equipment such as cardiac monitors and infusion pumps, have to be used anywhere in a hospital and must therefore have a standard mains plug. Standard mains socket outlets on the anaesthetic machine or intensive care ventilators or emergency trolleys are useful to the clinician, but an unrestricted number could lead to unacceptably high leakage currents. They would normally be used with equipment complying with IEC 601-1 and so the problem of leakage currents is considered to be of little importance for up to four auxiliary mains socket outlets. This number is a compromise between the benefits of several sockets against the incremental risk of exceeding tolerable leakage current.

It follows that the fitting of mains dividers or unauthorised equipment into these sockets can produce dangerous leakage currents. Many operating theatres and intensive care units have an insufficient number of power outlets and so there is a great temptation to break these rules.

Equipment other than emergency trolleys, anaesthetic work stations, and intensive care ventilators is not allowed to have any standard mains sockets.

Modern anaesthetic work stations, intensive care ventilators, and monitoring devices require electrical power to function normally. In the event of failure of the power supply there must be a power failure alarm (both for electrical and pneumatic power). Mains switches should also be provided with means to prevent inadvertent operation.

Certain types of equipment may be used in environments in which a defibrillator may be used and defibrillator protection is therefore required. After defibrillator discharge, the equipment is not only expected to remain safe but to function normally.

Electromagnetic interference is a serious design consideration with monitors. Interference may occur through the sensor, the sensor line, the monitor or its mains lead. It is difficult to control this interference but well designed monitors display clearly that interference renders the reading unreliable and return to normal action without recalibration. Electrocautery, mobile telephones, and more powerful electromagnets cause interference. A standard on this subject is being developed. Software errors are also a cause of concern and standards on this are also being developed.

Checklists for anaesthetic machines

In discussing the prevention of accidents with anaesthetic apparatus in 1968, Ward stressed that accidents can be prevented by:

- The thorough checking of anaesthetic equipment immediately before use
- Constant observation (by the anaesthetist) during anaesthesia
- An adequate knowledge of the structure and function of anaesthetic machines.[26]

Since that time machines have become more complex and the number of monitors has increased. Most assessments of the new generation of anaesthetic machines stress that their complexity means that anaesthetists should be thoroughly trained in their use before being allowed to use them on patients. This training should include a specific preuse checklist for the equipment. Manufacturers will also be required to provide a checklist to satisfy the proposed European standards on – for example, anaesthetic work stations.

Formal checklists have been developed by several national anaesthetic associations including the Association of Anaesthetists of Great Britain and Ireland and these should be used in concert with the checklist recommended by the machine manufacturer.[18] It is regrettable that this formal preuse checklist was only developed after serious accidents with machines which could have been prevented by a proper preuse checklist. Failure to perform a preuse check is a failure of 18% to 33% of mortality related to anaesthetic equipment or major failures.[27-30]

The Association of Anaesthetists incorporated the ideas suggested by the Faculty of Anaesthetists of the Royal Australasian College of Surgeons in 1980 in which checks of gases, rotameters, vaporisers, pre-circuit leaks, breathing system selection, circle system, were listed for easy memory.[31] The checklist is designed to be done in a few minutes and in practice takes from five to 19 minutes (mean 8·9).[20] Its features are listed in box 5. The recommended tests should be adapted in hospitals as a questionnaire and formally completed every day; a record of the check should be

---

Box 5 – Features of preanaesthetic checklist

- Check that oxygen analyser on the machine detects incorrectly filled cylinders – for example, contamination of oxygen pipeline as well as pipeline cross over
- Check vaporiser mounting and gas or liquid leakage and back-bar pressure relief (adequate detection of gas leakage may require other tests)[32]
- Check integrity and configuration of breathing system, adjustable pressure limited (APL) valve function, and leakage from breathing system
- Check the operation of the ventilator and its controls, function of the pressure relief valves, disconnect valve and availability of an emergency ventilator or resuscitator
- Check suction equipment

---

kept. This format is given in the Appendix to the paper by Bartram and McClymont in which they reviewed their experience with this checklist.[20] The authors analysed 55 completed checklists and noted that no problems arose from equipment which had been missed by the checklist. Faults were found in 60% of machines and 18% of these were thought to be serious. The design of monitors should facilitate automatic checking when the monitor is turned on. Integrated monitors should be centrally activated through the mains switch.

Training with equipment

Anaesthetic machines, anaesthetic work stations, and intensive care ventilators are complex and varied in design and function. Manufacturers must supply such information as marking on the equipment and package, an "instruction for use" document for users, and a "technical description" of the equipment. The format and content of this information is specified in European standards, but the documents often get misplaced or are too complex to follow. It is wise to ask the manufacturer to demonstrate his machine in the theatre or intensive care unit in which it is to be used. A protocol for training on the equipment should be used to ensure that every anaesthetist has formally been instructed in its use before using it on patients. This is a legal requirement in Germany.

A disciplined policy for the selection, purchasing and maintenance schedule for all equipment is essential for its safe use. The Department of Health document "Health equipment information – management of medical equipment and devices", HEI 98, provides indispensable advice on this subject.[33]

1 *Medical gas cylinder, valves and yoke connections*. London: British Standards Institution, 1955:BS 1319.
2 *York type valve connections for small medical gas cylinders used for anaesthetic and resuscitation purposes*. Geneva: International Standards Organisation, 1964:ISO 407.
3 *Identification of medical gas cylinders*. Geneva: International Standards Organisation, 1977:ISO 32.
4 *Anaesthetic and analgesic machines. Part III Specification for continuous flow anaesthetic machines*. London: British Standards Institution, 1989:BS 4272.
5 *Anaesthetic machines for use with humans*. Geneva: International Standards Organisation, 1980:ISO 5358.
6 Schreiber P, Schreiber JM. *Electronic surveillance during anaesthesia*. Telford, PA: North American Dräger, 1986.
7 *Recommendations for standards of monitoring during anaesthesia and recovery*. London: Association of Anaesthetists of Great Britain and Ireland, 1988.
8 Desmonts J-M, Duncan PG. A perspective on studies of anaesthesia morbidity and mortality. *Eur J Anaesthesiol* 1993;**10**(Suppl 7):33–41.
9 Allnutt MF. Human factors in accidents. *Br J Anaesth* 1987;**59**:856–64.
10 *Safety of medical electrical equipment*. 2nd edition. 1988:IEC 601-1.
11 Sugg R. Sound the alarm on signals standard. *Inside Healthcare* 1991;Sept:7–8.
12 Kestin IG, Miller BR, Lockhart CH. Auditory alarms during anaesthesia monitoring. *Anesthesiology* 1988;**69**:106–9.
13 *Low pressure flexible connecting assemblies (hose assemblies) for use with medical gas systems*. Geneva: International Standards Organisation, 1989:ISO 5359.
14 Abraham ZA, Basagiota J. A potentially lethal anaesthetic machine failure. *Anesthesiology* 1987;**66**:589–90.
15 *Anaesthetic machines for use with humans*. Geneva: International Standards Organisation, 1992:ISO 5358.
16 Michon-Bayer-Chammard F, Fischier M, Douau PY, Vourch G. Hypoxia due to failure of oxygen with nitrous oxide. *Ann Fr Anesth Reanim* 1988;**7**:165–8.
17 Schreiber P. *Safety guidelines for anesthesia systems*. Telford, PA: North American Dräger.
18 *Checklist for anaesthetic machines. A recommended procedure based on the use of an oxygen analyser*. London: Association of Anaesthetists of Great Britain and Ireland, 1990.
19 Merilainen PT. A differential sensor for breath-by-breath oximetry. *J Clin Monit* 1989;**6**:65–73.
20 Bartram C, McClymont W. The use of a checklist for anaesthetic machines. *Anaesthesia* 1992;**47**:1066–9.
21 Anaesthetic and respiratory equipment – conical connectors. Part 1: cones and sockets. Geneva: International Standards Organisation, 1987:ISO 5356-1.
22 *Anaesthetic and respiratory equipment – Part 2: screw-threaded weight bearing connectors*. Geneva: International Standards Organisation, 1987:ISO 5356-2.
23 Sykes MK. Essential monitoring. *Br J Anaesth* 1987;**9**:901–12.
24 *Anaesthetic reservoir bags*. Geneva: International Standards Organisation, 1980:ISO 5362.
25 *Inhalational breathing systems – Part 2. Anaesthetic circle breathing systems*. Geneva: International Standards Organisation, 1983:ISO 8835-2.
26 Ward C. The prevention of accidents associated with anaesthetic apparatus. *Br J Anaesth* 1968;**40**:692–701.
27 Craig J, Wilson ME. A survey of anaesthetic misadventures. *Anaesthesia* 1981;**36**:933–6.
28 Cooper JB, Newbower RS, Kitz RJ. An analysis of major errors and equipment failure in anesthesia: management considerations for prevention and detection. *Anesthesiology* 1984;**60**:30–42.
29 Lunn JN, Mushin WW. *Mortality associated with anaesthesia*. London: Nuffield Provincial Hospitals Trust, 1982.
30 *Report of a survey of anaesthetic practice*. London: Association of Anaesthetists of Great Britain and Ireland, 1988.

31 Faculty Documents T2. Protocol for checking an anaesthetic machine before use. *Royal Australasian College of Surgeons Bulletin* 1984;4:32.
32 Jackson IJB, Wilson RJT. Association of Anaesthetists' checklist for anaesthetic machines. Problems with significant leaks. *Anaesthesia* 1993;**48**:152–3.
33 *Health equipment information management of medical equipment and devices.* London: Department of Health, 1990:HEI 98.

10 Monitoring in anaesthesia

R F ARMSTRONG

During the last decade the number of techniques for monitoring patients during anaesthesia has increased considerably. This process, the result of a natural search for improvement in medical care, has to a lesser extent been driven by a desire to avoid expensive litigation.[1] In particular the concept of minimal monitoring introduced by hospitals associated with Harvard Medical School has attracted widespread interest and application.

What is the mortality and morbidity associated with anaesthesia?

Estimates of the death rate caused by anaesthesia vary. One of the first reviews suggested that the rate was about 3/10 000 anaesthetics,[2] but more recently the Confidential Enquiry into Perioperative Deaths (CEPOD) carried out in the United Kingdom reported 4000 deaths in three health regions in over half a million anaesthetics.[3] Of these, three (0·1%) were the direct result of anaesthesia and in 72 (1·8%) the anaesthetic was contributory. The death rate of 0·054/10 000 anaesthetics calculated in the British study compares favourably with other reports. Eichhorn from the Beth Israel Hospital and Harvard Medical School reported a death rate of 0·066/10 000 from 1976–85,[4] and an older French study (1978–82) described a rate of 0·76/10 000.[5]

In addition to deaths there are of course other injuries caused by anaesthesia, particularly brain damage. In an editorial on vegetative survival after brain injuries, Jennett drew attention to studies from two medical defence societies in the United Kingdom indicating a "substantial incidence of claims for severe brain damage" of which 70% had been associated with anaesthesia.[6] It is difficult to establish the true extent of this morbidity. The data from the medical defence societies (including doctors and dentists from the United Kingdom and Australasia) have suggested there is a case of severe cerebral damage every month. In a recent survey, the Quality of Practice Committee collected 169 cases of unintentional cardiac arrest or events leading to brain damage occurring within six hours of anaesthesia during a 12 month period.[7] Of these, 55 were clearly related to anaesthesia though the population at risk was not established.

Given the study period of 30 postoperative days used by CEPOD, Jennett pointed out that this will fail to capture most brain damaged patients and made a plea for audit to include serious complications and "near misses."

What are the causes of anaesthetic accidents?

Cooper et al defined critical incidents[11] as a human error or equipment failure that could have led (if not discovered or corrected in time) or did lead to an undesirable outcome, ranging from increased length of hospital stay to death.[8 21] In a survey of 1089 such incidents he concluded that disconnection of the breathing circuit, swapping of syringes, and problems with gas flow were the main causes. Human error was a factor in 80% of cases.

Keenan and Bayan reviewed 27 anaesthesia related cardiac arrests and showed that in 11 cases there was "failure to ventilate."[9] In a closed claims study from the United States 193 of 624 claims resulted from "respiratory mishaps" including 80 from inadequate ventilation and 41 from oesophageal intubation.[10] In 1989 Eichhorn et al analysed 11 major intraoperative accidents caused solely by anaesthesia (five deaths, four cases of permanent neurological damage, and two cardiac arrests).[11] They concluded that "unrecognised hypoventilation is the commonest intraoperative anaesthesia accident leading to severe patient injury" and that disconnection of components of the breathing system was the most common anaesthesia related mishap. Evidence of human error abounds. Inadequate preanaesthetic assessment, poor supervision of inexperienced anaesthetists, and inadequate monitoring were features of the CEPOD report.[3] In the United States, failure to monitor, poor preoperative assessment, absence from theatre, and inadequate supervision of recovery were responsible for over half the successful claims. Chopra *et al* reported failure to check, lack of vigilance, and carelessness.[12] Anaesthetic apparatus has also often been criticised for its great age and lack of user friendliness.

Response of the profession

Against this background of accident and death, how has the profession responded? A key initiative was made by the Boston hospitals attached to the Harvard Medical School. This was followed by the introduction of minimal monitoring standards by the American Society of Anesthesiologists in 1985. These standards have been steadily upgraded since and currently 12 countries have adopted minimal monitoring standards. That they are welcomed by the insurers is clear; lower premiums for anaesthetists have already been introduced in some areas. In New York certain standards have become law. In the United Kingdom the Association of Anaesthetists have published an important document on monitoring.[13] Though the document consists of recommendations, Taylor and Goldhill make the point that this document will inevitably be used by the courts to define the profession's minimum standards.[14]

Summary of main recommendations of Association of Anaesthetists

(a) The anaesthetist should be present throughout the conduct of the whole anaesthetic and should ensure that an adequate record of the procedure is made.

(b) Monitoring should be commenced before induction of anaesthesia and continued until the patient has recovered from the anaesthetic.

(c) Monitoring of anaesthetic machine function should include an oxygen analyser (with alarms) and devices which enable leaks, disconnections, rebreathing or overpressure of the breathing system to be detected.

(d) *Continuous* monitoring of ventilation and circulation is essential. This may be performed by use of the human senses augmented, where appropriate, by the use of monitoring equipment. *Clinical observations* include the patient's colour, responses to the surgical stimulus, movements of the chest wall and reservoir bag, palpation of the pulse and auscultation of the breath and heart sounds. *Continuous* monitoring devices include the pulse plethysmograph, the pulse oximeter, the electrocardiograph, the capnograph, and devices for measuring vascular pressures and body temperature.

175

(e) When intermittent non-invasive methods are used to measure arterial pressure and heart rate the frequency of measurement should be appropriate to the clinical state of the patient.

(f) A peripheral nerve stimulator should be readily available when neuromuscular blocking drugs are employed.

(g) Additional monitoring may be required for long or complicated operations and for patients with co-existing medical disease.

(h) Adequate monitoring is needed during brief anaesthetics or when using local anaesthetic or sedation techniques which may lead to loss of consciousness or to cardiovascular or respiratory complications.

(i) Appropriate monitoring should also be used during transport of the patient.

(j) Anaesthetists should issue clear instructions concerning monitoring of postoperative care when handing over the patient to recovery ward staff. Appropriate monitoring facilities should be available in the recovery ward.

Recommended monitoring techniques: instruments

Amongst the important recommendations made in this document are a key group of monitoring instruments.[13]

Oxygen analyser

This instrument is of fundamental importance to the checklist for anaesthetic machines proposed by the Association of Anaesthetists of Great Britain and Ireland.[15] Paramagnetic oxygen analysers, as used in the Datex gas analysis monitor, depend on the fact that oxygen molecules are attracted by magnets. They are accurate and respond rapidly to changing concentrations. Polarographic analysers on the other hand function electrochemically. In the Clark type (Ohmeda 5120 oxygen monitor) a cathode responds to the presence of oxygen in solution by generating a current proportional to its concentration. The analyser consumes some oxygen and usually responds slowly. The membrane has to be changed regularly. Fuel cell analysers function in the same way though an internal chemical reaction provides the electronic potential rather than a battery.

When monitors that sample gas are used, some thought has to be given to disposal of the gas. If it is returned to the breathing circuit there may be a danger of contamination. In low flow closed circuit anaesthesia, continuous sampling can result in appreciable loss of the volume of gases. These considerations apart, oxygen analysers will detect changes in oxygen concentration (though not flow) when placed distal to the common gas outlet and as close to the patient as possible. Some authors have suggested that the analyser should be placed in the expiratory limb so that the alarms would be activated by the low expired oxygen concentration if low flow developed inadvertently.[14]

Setting the alarm just below the desired inspired oxygen concentration has been recommended for inspiratory limb oxygen analysers to give the anaesthetist time to respond to any reduction in oxygen flow.[16] An upper limit of 40% in oxygen concentration will identify any failure in the nitrous oxide supply.

Disconnection and high pressure alarms

Although pulmonary damage may occur at any airway pressure, pneumothorax is more common at pressures above 40 cm of water, so high pressure alarms will warn against lung damage as well as indicating blockage or compression of the delivery tubing. Disconnection alarms are triggered by failure to reach a given pressure and some thought must be given to the alarm setting. In the event that there is *some* circuit resistance, an appreciable positive pressure may be maintained throughout the respiratory cycle even in the presence of a dangerous leak. For this reason low pressure alarms of about 1·2 kPa have been recommended by some authorities.[17]

Continuous monitoring of ventilation and circulation

The pulse oximeter has become widely accepted, world sales in 1989 being estimated at 65 000 units. A recent review of pulse oximetry included 249 references, which indicates the interest shown by the profession.[18] The function of a pulse oximeter is based on the transmission of two wavelengths of 660 nm (red) and 940 nm (infrared) from a light emitting diode. When these bands of light are directed across a finger or ear-lobe they are sensed by photodiodes which produce a current depending on the quantity of light absorbed. Light absorbed by the non-pulsatile tissues (tissue bed, venous blood, capillary blood, and non-pulsatile arterial blood), which is sometimes referred to as the direct current or baseline component, is subtracted from the total signal. This yields the absorption produced by the pulsatile arteriolar bed or the alternating current signal.

Absorption in the blood is by oxyhaemoglobin (HbO_2) and its

177

congenors, carboxyhaemoglobin (HbCO), reduced haemoglobin (Hb), and methaemoglobin (MetHb). As pulse oximeters have only two wavelengths they do not differentiate among all these species. The presence of carboxyhaemoglobin is "seen" by the oximeter as oxyhaemoglobin. Methaemoglobin, which has almost the same absorbance as reduced haemoglobin, causes the oximeter to record low figures incorrectly when the actual arterial oxygen saturation is high. These additional haemoglobins have resulted in the introduction of the terms "functional haemoglobin saturation" ($HBO_2/HbO_2 + Hb \times 100\%$) and "fractional haemoglobin saturation" ($HbO_2/HbO_2 + Hb + COHb + MetHb \times 100\%$). When methaemoglobin and carboxyhaemoglobin are present four wavelengths would be needed to measure functional or fractional haemoglobin saturation.[19]

Other limitations include under–reading during severe vasoconstriction, motion artefact, and interference by ambient light. False alarms, most often caused by motion, can create such irritation that the attendant is driven to disarm the instrument. Accuracy at higher levels of arterial oxygen saturation is generally good. A more worrying problem is the slow response to deteriorating pulmonary function when high concentrations of oxygen are given. On 60% oxygen even a patient with poor respiratory function may achieve an arterial oxygen tension of – for example, 30 kPa. Even if respiratory function worsens, the saturation will not begin to fall until the arterial oxygen tension reaches 10 kPa. In these circumstances the oximeter has been compared to a road sign placed at the top of a cliff, and only visible to the occupants of a car as they plunge over the edge.[19]

End tidal carbon dioxide monitoring

Monitoring the concentration or partial pressure of carbon dioxide by the absorption of infrared radiation in the inspired and expired gas mixture has provided the anaesthetist with yet more insight into the patient's respiratory and metabolic state.

Using this capnographic technique, respiratory problems (underventilation, oesophageal intubation), metabolic disorders (hyperpyrexia), malfunction of machines (leak and disconnection), and even circulatory changes (cardiac arrest or embolism) can be detected. It is small wonder that this instrument has proved to be so popular in modern anaesthetic practice. The capnogram produced shows a characteristic shape which was described by

Gravenstein *et al* as an elephant swallowed by a snake.[16] Distortions of shape occur with various clinical abnormalities and are summarised in fig.1.

One of the most useful applications of end tidal capnography is that it detects disconnection, obstruction, or inadvertent oesophageal intubation by recording a zero or near zero end tidal carbon dioxide reading. An acute fall in end tidal carbon dioxide generally indicates a serious or dramatic event. It may represent pulmonary embolus by clot, fragment, or air, or sudden hypotension as a result of haemorrhage. A more gradual decrease suggests a progressive increase in the alveolar to arterial carbon dioxide gradient caused by an increase in dead space. This may be caused by excessive positive end expiratory pressure (PEEP) or by a fall in cardiac output.

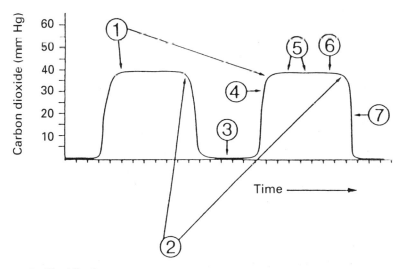

FIG 1—Checklist for a capnogram:
1 Plateau/onset: Is there a pattern giving evidence of ventilation?
2 Plateau/peak: Are peak values appropriate? Are the ventilator settings and the patient's respiratory pattern consistent with the capnogram and capnographic findings?
3 Baseline: Is the inspired carbon dioxide tension zero (normal baseline), or is there evidence of rebreathing (raised baseline)?
4 Upstroke: Is there evidence of slow exhalation (slanted upstroke)?
5 Plateau/horizontal: Is there evidence of uneven emptying of lungs?
6 Plateau/smooth: Is expiration interrupted by inspiratory efforts?
7 Downstroke: Is the downstroke steep, or is there evidence of slow inspiration or partial rebreathing?

As with other instruments it pays to recognise limitations. If there is a ventilation/perfusion mismatch, the end tidal carbon dioxide may be appreciably lower than the arterial tension. Sampling techniques (sidestream sampling, low sampling flow rates, filters, and long sampling lines) may result in delayed responses, damping, incorrect values, and a lack of synchronisation between the machine and the actual respiratory cycle. Where should the alarm limits be set? Low arterial carbon dioxide tension may result in impaired cerebral blood flow. If the capnograph is expected to report this as well as acute dead space disorders (air embolism), a lower alarm limit of 3·0 kPa may be considered necessary. This will also report disconnection and apnoea. A high alarm set at 7·0 kPa will draw attention to hypoventilation, though this may be too high for neurosurgical techniques. Many capnometers also monitor respiratory rate and can therefore be armed accordingly.

In a study of 11 major intraoperative accidents in 1 001 000 anaesthetics, Eichhorn et al concluded that eight could have been prevented by safety monitoring.[11] Capnography would have been the most useful method, followed by oximetry.

Electrocardiography

The benefits of electrocardiography include the detection of arrhythmias, alterations in heart rate, and in some cases the ability to recognise ischaemia by changes in the ST segment. As with all monitors, setting of the alarms is recommended (fig 2).

Attempts to recognise operative ischaemia were the stimulus for the introduction of the CM5 lead. In this configuration the left arm lead is placed in the V5 position (left fifth intercostal space in the anterior axillary line), the right arm lead on the central manubrium, and the indifferent lead on the left shoulder. One of the most common signs of ischaemia is ST depression, usually shown in the lateral leads. More recently it has been recognised that diagnostic accuracy is increased if multilead monitoring is used.[20] The selection of leads that offers the best chance of detecting ischaemia is controversial. Some authorities consider V4 and V5 to be the most sensitive. That uncertainty surrounds the optimal form of electrocardiographic monitoring is highlighted by a recent report of the failure of Holter monitoring to detect an acute operative myocardial infarction which was clearly seen on the 12 lead electrocardiogram.[21] Given the growing prevalence of cardiovascular disease and an ageing population, more focused use of the

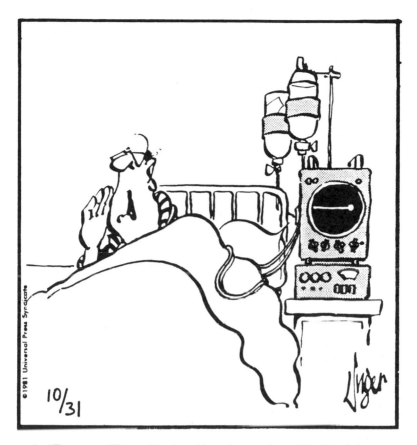

FIG 2—"Excuse me. The machine is making a funny noise and the little light is going in a straight line."

electrocardiogram during the operation is becoming increasingly important.

Mangano, in a comprehensive review of American practice, makes the point that perioperative cardiac morbidity is the leading cause of death after anaesthesia and operation.[22] Preoperative predictors of poor outcome are previous myocardial infarction, congestive heart failure, hypertension, diabetes, and peripheral vascular disease. These and operative factors like an emergency operation, vascular surgery, and prolonged thoracic or upper abdominal surgery mean that extra efforts must be made to detect myocardial ischaemia. In these cases multiple lead electrocardiography may be more sensitive than the standard three lead system. There is increasing evidence that the danger of myocardial ischaemia is greater in the postoperative period than during the relatively controlled stage of supervised anaesthesia. Attention is now being directed to this area of care.

Invasive monitoring

Blood pressure

The need for beat to beat blood pressure measurement in certain clinical circumstances has led to the increasingly popular procedure of arterial catheterisation, but the technique has its drawbacks. Anyone who approaches a patient for the first time with intent to puncture would be well advised to read Bedford's definitive chapter on the subject before proceeding.[23]

Indications for arterial monitoring include the need for intensive care, cardiothoracic surgery, hypotensive anaesthesia, or surgery involving serious blood loss, together with unstable, high risk patients and those who required regular blood gas monitoring.

Insertion

Most authorities now recommend the use of Teflon catheters because of their reduced potential to thrombose. Small catheters (20–22 gauge) should be preferred though they are more prone to kink. They are associated with a lower incidence of blockage of vessels and show good pressure transmission characteristics. With continuous slow flush by a heparinised solution, good nursing care, and attention to sterility these catheters may last indefinitely. Most workers recognise, however, that colonisation rates start to increase at 96 hours and several groups recommend changing to a new site at this stage.[24] Other indications for change include evidence of ischaemia, suspected infection, and blood cultures that grow pathogens. Distal sites in the lower extremities should usually be avoided because of the high incidence of thrombosis and the pronounced augmentation of systolic pressure that occurs. The reputation of the femoral arteries as being a "dirty" area has recently been refuted. Certainly when poor access, shock, or burns make radial catheterisation difficult the femoral artery can provide a safe haven.

Monitoring instrumentation

Once the arterial cannula is in place, connection can be made to a fluid filled line and transducer. When setting the transducer to zero, the reference point is usually taken from the level of the right atrium (fourth intercostal space in the midaxillary line) when the patient is supine. The importance of excluding bubbles and avoiding excessive lengths of tubing are crucial if the displayed pressure is to bear any relation to reality.

What reality actually is, in terms of blood pressure, is difficult to define. Certainly the systolic pressure displayed on the screen can be misleading. Several points are worth mentioning. Direct invasive pressure measurement does not agree with indirect cuff measurement, which relies on flow past the cuff. Peripheral artery traces generally show higher systolic values than those from the aorta. This augmentation is the result of reflection of the pulse pressure wave at the artery/arteriole junction and resonance of the wave caused by the physical characteristics of the connecting system. As a result systolic pressure does not equal aortic arch pressure. Mean pressure generally does. Finally it should be remembered that peripheral systolic pressure does not equate with flow.

Choice of artery

Though axillary, brachial, and femoral arteries are all legitimate sites in which to insert cannulas, it is the radial artery which is the clinician's usual target. Bedford makes the comment: "It would seem imprudent to cannulate a radial artery in a hand with inadequate ulnar artery collateral circulation". How one achieves verification of an adequate collateral flow is controversial. Bedford occludes the artery with one finger and feels for a distal retrograde pulse with another. The modified Allen test has not satisfied all workers, and several other techniques including Doppler examination, plethysmography and pulse oximetry have been proposed.[25] Digital ischaemia resulting in amputation has been reported, and may start with blockage of the catheter. Attempts to fast flush blocked catheters may cause retrograde flow of flush solution bubbles, or fragments of clot, as far as the cerebral circulation. It is clear that at the first sign of ischaemia the catheter should be removed.

Central venous pressure

Though it is slightly unfashionable, central venous pressure measurement has an important place in the armamentarium of the modern anaesthetist. Its main virtue lies in its safety and simplicity, and an understanding of its failings developed over the years. Right atrial pressure is a more practical way of assessing preload than myocardial fibre length or right ventricular end diastolic volume. It allows insight into venous return and so helps to assess cardiac function and intravascular volume.

Central venous pressure measured from the midaxillary line usually lies between 5–10 mm Hg (multiply by 1·36 to convert measurement to cm of water). It should be measured at the end of expiration. A single measurement can, however, be misleading. The relation between pressure and volume is not linear in the heart or the vascular bed and is affected by changes in the compliance of either system. For this reason the response of the central venous pressure to a fluid challenge is a much more useful approach. If the volume of the vascular space is in question, a fluid challenge of 200 ml colloid may provoke a transient rise and rapid fall in central venous pressure suggestive of underfilling. A sustained rise with only slow return to baseline suggests overfilling or an uncompliant ventricle.

Insertion and management

There are several approaches to the central veins in common use, and clinicians should become familiar with all of them. Whichever entry is chosen, scrupulous asepsis is necessary. Once the catheter is in place, blood should be aspirated through it. At the earliest opportunity a radiograph should be taken to verify that the position is correct and to exclude pneumothorax. Opinions vary on how long to leave central venous catheters in place. In critically ill patients the incidence of catheter related sepsis increases with time, and many centres advise changing catheters at regular intervals (seven days), but a recent survey concluded that changing catheters at specified intervals was probably unnecessary.[24] It was considered better to change when there was a clinical indication (such as infection at the site or signs of catheter-related sepsis). In these circumstances there is support for the technique of guide wire exchange followed by culture of the removed catheter and subsequent change to a new catheter and new site if the removed one is contaminated.

Pulmonary artery catheterisation

In patients with heart failure, hypotension, or severe hypoxaemia who are unresponsive to normal resuscitative measures, a useful guide to treatment is the measurement of pulmonary artery wedge pressure. This technique has recently been recommended by the American Society of Anesthesiologists for operative use in patients at increased risk of haemodynamic disturbance.[26] These are patients with cardiovascular disease, pulmonary dysfunction, renal insufficiency and advanced age; as well as sepsis, burns, and trauma. In these cases a pulmonary artery catheter should be inserted before operation. From this procedure information can be gained about left ventricular preload (affecting stroke volume), pulmonary venous pressure (affecting extravascular lung water), and pulmonary vascular resistance (affecting right ventricular function). If a catheter incorporating a thermodilution probe is used, cardiac output[27] and stroke volume can be measured as well., This will give more insight into cardiovascular dynamics than with wedge pressure alone. As with right atrial pressure, individual readings are of less value than responses to fluid challenges, inotropes, or vasodilators.

Dangers of pulmonary artery catheterisation

Dangers are appreciable and aseptic technique is important. During advancement of the catheter, arrhythmias are common and it is important not to insert more than 15–20 cm without seeing a change in chamber pressure. This will avoid coiling and knotting. Once the catheter is in position, care must be taken to avoid it persistently wedging in a small pulmonary vessel. Overinflation of the balloon which may cause vascular damage and haemoptysis has also been reported. Accuracy is increased by taking the measurement at end exhalation and by attending to transducer preparation.

It is important to appreciate the limitations of measuring pulmonary artery wedge pressure. Under certain circumstances (such as positive end expiratory pressure, high airway pressure, or hypotension) the discrepancy between pulmonary artery wedge pressure and left atrial pressure may increase. The same problem occurs if the catheter tip is placed in a poorly perfused part of the lung. Of crucial importance is to realise that a stiff and uncompliant ventricle will cause further divergence between atrial pressure and ventricular volume. In these circumstances pulmonary artery wedge pressure may be a poor guide to the amount of fluid

185

that is required. In low output states, judicious fluid challenges and repeated estimation of stroke volume with construction of ventricular function curves is a better way of planning a strategy than a reliance on pressure. As soon as the necessary information is obtained and the patient stable the catheter should be removed.

Is modern monitoring minimal, maximal, or (maybe) misdirected?

In the dash for increasingly comprehensive monitoring, a few questioning voices have been heard. Orkin pointed to the problem of limited funds, demands for services exceeding the ability of society to pay for them, and the danger of consuming other people's resources.[28] From an epidemiological standpoint it is possible in the United Kingdom to question the view that anaesthesia represents a serious public health challenge. Using the CEPOD figures for three health regions studied, there were only three deaths in one year from a population of roughly 10 million. Crude extrapolation suggests an annual total for the United Kingdom of 18 deaths, compared with 180 000 deaths from heart disease and 19 000 from cancer of the large bowel.[29]

When looked at from this perspective it is clear that any extra spending must be justified if there is to be net benefit. The costs are high. Investing in 10 instruments capable of recording oxygen saturation, capnography, electrocardiography, pressure and temperature would cost an average anaesthetic department in the United Kingdom about £100 000.

A reduction in litigation might offset this outlay. Eichhorn et al in their analysis of over a million patients cared for over a period of eight years by the Harvard department of anaesthesia, estimated the insurance loss for the 11 accidents he described as $5 391 000.[11] They also estimated that minimal operative monitoring would have prevented eight of these accidents and saved $4 756 000 during the period of the study for the nine component hospitals.

What is the evidence that monitoring will reduce morbidity and mortality? Given the rarity of an "anaesthetic" death, huge numbers of patients randomised to groups with and without monitoring would be needed to prove the point. In a retrospective analysis Eichhorn et al compared two groups of patients before and after the introduction of minimal monitoring. From 1976–85 757 000 patients were studied, and there were 10 accidents and five deaths.

From 1985 (and the introduction of standards) there was one accident and no deaths among 244 000 patients. Unfortunately, as Orkin pointed out, this difference is not significant and even if it was it could not be attributed to the introduction of monitoring. There was no control group and many other changes in both technique and training occurred during the period.

Keenan and Boyan also compared two periods of anaesthetic practice before and after the introduction of monitoring standards.[9] From 1969–83 there were 27 anaesthesia related cardiac arrests and 14 deaths in 163 240 cases. After adoption of monitoring standards there were none in a subsequent series of 25 000 patients. This study is continuing. More recent efforts to show the benefits of monitoring have shown a fall in unanticipated admissions to the intensive care unit since the introduction of oximetry.[30] These apparent improvements from retrospective studies have to be set against the already reported trend towards lower accident rates before the introduction of intensive monitoring.

In a report from South Africa covering the years 1956–87, Harrison described a fall in anaesthetic mortality from 0·43/1000 in the first five years to 0·07/1000 anaesthetics in the last five years.[31] Finally, in a rare controlled and prospective trial Moller et al from Denmark failed to show any reduction in postoperative complications after the introduction of oximetry though more episodes of desaturation were detected and the incidence of angina and ST segment depression was reduced.[32 33]

However, it is not just anaesthetic deaths that we are intent on reducing but overall morbidity and mortality. Recent studies have suggested that anaesthesia may be indirectly responsible for more deaths than have hitherto been suspected.[34] Newer monitoring tools such as the oesophageal Doppler and the tonometer can predict postoperative complications and have emphasised the importance of inadequate circulation in the pathogenesis of postoperative problems. Perhaps we need to focus on which monitoring is best. Norman, during a symposium on "Mishap or negligence" at the Royal College of Anaesthetists, concluded that the use of routine minimal monitoring as a routine had much to commend it. Most patients would agree.

1 Cohen MM, Wade J, Woodward C. Medicolegal concerns among Canadian anaesthetists. *Can J Anaesth* 1990;37:102–11.
2 Beecher HK, Todd DP. A study of the deaths associated with anaesthesia and surgery based on a study of 599428 anaesthesias in 10 institutions 1948–1952 inclusive. *Ann Surg* 1954;140:2–35.

3 Buck N, Devlin HB, Lunn JN. *Report of a confidential enquiry into perioperative deaths.* London: Nuffield Provincial Trust and King's Fund, 1987.

4 Eichhorn JH. Prevention of intraoperative anaesthesia accidents and related severe injury through safety monitoring. *Anesthesiology* 1989;70:572–7.

5 Tiret L, Desmonts JM, Hatton F, Vourc'h G. Complications associated with anaesthesia – a prospective survey in France. *Can Anaesth Soc J* 1986;33:336–44.

6 Jennett B. Vegetative survival after brain insults, can anaesthetists reduce the frequency of a fate worse than death? *Anaesthesia* 1988;43:921–2.

7 Stoddart JC. *Register of brain damage/cardiac arrests.* Quality of Practice Committee. London: Royal College of Anaesthetists, 1993.

8 Cooper JB, Newbower RS, Kitz RJ. An analysis of major errors and equipment failures in anesthesia management: considerations for prevention and detection. *Anesthesiology* 1984;60:34–42.

9 Keenan RL, Boyan CP. Cardiac arrests due to anaesthesia. A study of incidence and causes. *JAMA* 1985;253:2373–7.

10 Cheney FW, Posner K, Caplan RA, Ward RJ. Standards of care and anesthesia liability. *JAMA* 1989;261:1599–603.

11 Eichhorn JH, Cooper JB, Cullen DJ, Maier WR, Philip JH, Seeman RG. Standards of patient monitoring during anaesthesia at Harvard Medical School. *JAMA* 1986;256:1017–20.

12 Chopra V, Bovill JG, Spierdijk J?. Accidents, near accidents and complications during anaesthesia. A retrospective analysis of a 10 year period in a teaching hospital. *Anaesthesia* 1990;45:3–6.

13 *Recommendations for standards of monitoring during anaesthesia and recovery.* London: Association of Anaesthetists of Great Britain and Ireland, 1988.

14 Taylor TH, Goldhill DR. *Standards of care in anaesthesia.* Butterworth – Heinemann, 1992.

15 *Checklist for anaesthetic machines.* London: Association of Anaesthetists of Great Britain and Ireland, 1990.

16 Gravenstein JS, Paulus DA, Hayes TJ. Capnography in clinical practice. Stoneham, Butterworth, 1989.

17 Pryne SJ, Cross MM. Ventilator disconnection alarm failure. *Anaesthesia* 1989;44:978–81.

18 Severinghaus JW, Kelleher JF. Recent developments in pulse oximetry. *Anesthesiology* 1992;76:1018–38.

19 Tremper KK, Barker SJ. Pulse oximetry. *Anesthesiology* 1989;70:98–108.

20 London MJ, Hollenberg M, Wong MG, Levenson L, Tubau JF, Browner W, *et al.* Intraoperative myocardial ischemia; localisation by continuous 12 lead electrocardiography. *Anesthesiology* 1988;69:232–41.

21 Marsh SCU, Castelli I, Schaefer HG, Skarvan K. Failure of continuous three channel Holter monitoring to detect acute perioperative myocardial infarction. *Anaesthesia* 1992;47:34–7.

22 Mangano DT. Perioperative cardiac morbidity. *Anesthesiology* 1990;72:153–84.

23 Bedford RF. Invasive blood pressure monitoring. In: Blitt CD, ed. *Monitoring in anaesthesia and critical care medicine.* 2nd ed. Edinburgh: Churchill Livingstone, 1990:93.

24 Norwood S, Ruby A, Civetta J, Cortes V. Catheter related infections and associated septicaemia. *Chest* 1991;99:968–75.

25 Fuhrman TM, Reilley TE, Pippin WD. Comparison of digital blood pressure, plethsmography, and the modified Allen's test as a means of evaluating the collateral circulation to the hand. *Anaesthesia* 1992;47:959–61.

26 American Society of Anesthesiologists Task Force on pulmonary artery catheterisation. Practice guidelines for pulmonary artery catheterisation. *Anesthesiology* 1993;78:380–94.

27 Nishikawa T, Dohi S. Errors in the measurement of cardiac output by thermodilution. *Can J Anaesth* 1993;40:142–53.

28 Orkin FR. Practice standards: the Midas touch or the emperor's new clothes? *Anesthesiology* 1989;70:567–71.

29 Jacobson B, Smith A, Whitehead M, eds. *The Nation's Health.* London: King Edward's Hospital Fund for London, 1991.

30 Cullen DJ, Nemaskal JR, Cooper JB, Zaslavsky A, Dwyer MJ. Effect of pulse oximetry, age, and ASA physical status on the frequency of patients admitted unexpectedly to a post-operative intensive care unit. *Anesth Analg* 1992;74:181–8.

31 Harrison GG. Deaths due to anaesthesia at Groote Schuur Hospital, Cape Town 1956–1987. *S Afr Med J* 1990;77:412–15.

32 Moller JT, Pederson T, Johannessen NW. Pulse oximetry does not reduce postoperative complications: a prospective study of 20802 patients. *Anesthesiology* 1991;**75**:A867.
33 Moller JT, Ravlo O, Jensen PF. Pulse oximetry uncovers hypoxemia and decreases the incidence of evidence for myocardial ischemia during anesthesia. *Anesthesiology* 1990;**75**:A1057.
34 Mythen MG, Webb AR. Intra-operative gut mucosal hypoperfusion is associated with increased post-operative complications and cost. *Intensive Care Med* 1994;**20**:99–104.

The summary of the main recommendations of the Association of Anaesthetists is reprinted with permission.

11 Managing a department of anaesthesia

ANN NAYLOR

Anaesthetic directorate

In 1988 the Association of Anaesthetists published a booklet entitled *Guidelines on duties of chairmen of divisions of anaesthesia*.[1] This stated that divisional chairmen, representing the specialty, accepted responsibility for organising the service and advising health authorities on all matters relating to anaesthetists and their delivery of care to patients. Since that time (with the NHS management changes, the development of resource management, and the introduction of purchaser/provider contracting) management structures based on clinical directorates have been introduced in many hospitals. Different units have evolved structures suited to their own requirements but underlying the changes has been the need for hospital resources to be managed by clinicians. This has led to the change from the division of anaesthesia to the clinical directorate with an important role in provider unit service delivery.

An anaesthetic directorate may hold the budgets for all anaesthetic services; the department of anaesthesia with all its staff, consultants and other career grades and trainees; the theatres and theatre staff; the pain service; resuscitation; obstetrics; the intensive care unit and its staff; even day surgery units, together with all the resources used there. At the other extreme, the budget for anaesthetists and their services may be held within other directorates, for example, general surgery, orthopaedics, or obstetrics and gynaecology. In the latter structure, anaesthetists may be involved in an advisory capacity from time to time but have no control of their own resources or future direction. Between these options other variations exist, but only by being in charge of their overall budget will anaesthetists be in control of the anaesthetic services in their hospital as recommended in a second booklet, *NHS management changes – implications for anaesthetists*.[2]

A strong clinical directorate has full budgetary responsibility. The involvement of a multi-disciplinary team is essential to run such a service; doctors, nurses, and managers all working together with shared aims and objectives. The typical management team for the directorate is clinical director, senior nurse manager, and business manager, and the nurse manager and business manager are appointed and managed by the clinical director who also sets their objectives and monitors their performance.

The clinical director has overall responsibility for organisation, strategic management, operational management, workload, and use of resources. Decisions about workload and quality standards, risk management issues, and business planning are shared by the management team with each having specific responsibilities. The nurse manager may be in charge of personnel issues, health and safety, risk management, and patient safety and satisfaction, and the business manager of information and finance.

Business managers are developing their roles as experience is gained within directorates, by providing costing services and financial and activity analysis, planning changes in delivery of services and monitoring progress against plans.

The anaesthetic directorate provides services to departments of surgery, to users of the intensive care and day units, and to some general practitioners through the pain clinic. It is a purchaser of drugs, equipment and services from departments such as central sterile supplies, the laundry, and the pharmacy. The quantity and quality of the service to be supplied within a given contract is crucial in all negotiations between purchaser and provider, and monitoring the quantity and quality of directorate services is essential.

The preparation of a business plan by the clinical director, the nurse manager and the business manager in which the current service provided, planning for future developments and changes in services, and establishing ways to maintain and develop the quality of service provision are defined is the main activity of the clinical directorate. The final business plan must be compatible with and part of the overall business plan of the unit. All staff in the directorate are affected by the business plan and obtaining some degree of acceptance and understanding of the new management processes has been important for their acceptability and success with all staff.

The clinical directorate requires support to achieve success. In physical terms this means appropriate accommodation and technology for business planning and gathering information. In terms of staff it means appropriate secretarial assistance and advice from a management accountant and a personnel officer.

Medical staff

Together with adequate professional representation, anaesthetists have some obligation for economy and efficiency (however distasteful this may seem). They will be seeking adequate anaesthetic cover for duties before, during, and after operations together with services to treat acute pain. They will have to help trainees with their training and accreditation; and they will need assistance in the operating theatre, the recovery departments, and in high dependency units. They will also need equipment and optimal standards of monitoring and they will need help with audit. This list also includes adequate arrangements for an obstetric service, for an emergency service, and intensive care and chronic pain services.

Anaesthetists recognise that their performance is set against their contracts and that these contracts will be monitored. They have not previously been professionally answerable to the chairman of the division of anaesthetics, but are now answerable through the clinical director to the medical director of the Trust for adequate performance. Each consultant has a job plan that is reviewed annually. Information on workload is required for budgetary apportionment of costs to surgical services and the job plans are needed for this and for the overall business plan of the directorate.

Clarifying and defining existing duties in the job plans will show which areas are funded and which not funded and the process of discussing and agreeing job plans can be used in establishing the case for additional consultants or negotiating alterations in work commitments.

Anaesthetic care has traditionally been organised departmentally in contrast to the medical and surgical consultant-led firms.

As the largest single specialty, anaesthetic directorates have the most consultant staff in most provider units. Each consultant has been used to having full clinical freedom and autonomy and each finds changes difficult to accept.

It is usual to distribute responsibilities among clinicians in the department, leaving one clinician as professional chairman who is responsible for the overall direction of medical staff, anaesthetic staff recruitment and retention, teaching and training, accreditation, study leave, recognition and research. Other clinicians are responsible for subdirectorates such as relief of chronic pain, obstetric services, tutor in anaesthetics, and Association of Anaesthetists linkman.

The attitudes of others to the anaesthetic department such as surgeons, physicians, other clinical directors, and the chief executive and Trust Board depend on the style of representation of the directorate of anaesthesia. It is important that all the anaesthetists work together and consult together about service development, contract pricing, volume setting, and quality specifications.

Subdirectorates

Subdirectorates can be set up within a large directorate – for instance, intensive care, maternity services, pain services, or the day unit. The key requirement for a subdirectorate is that the clinician in charge takes over the resource management and budget for the area and is involved in its business planning.

The primary need is for a clinician "with an interest" in the area and an established clinical credibility. Being prepared to work with colleagues in the subdirectorates and to cooperate with the clinical director is essential as management accountability will be involved. Such a clinician can develop and monitor the use of management protocols, admission criteria, and audit. Business plans can be developed for each subdirectorate and built into the directorate business plan as that plan in turn is built into the overall business plan of the organisation. Areas such as intensive care (which is not a typical ward and has many difficult ethical, clinical, and management problems), and areas which are not "ward-based" (such as maternity services and pain services) need such clinical leaders. To achieve this type of management each clinician will require some office space, secretarial assistance, and backing from the senior nurse manager and business manager of the directorate. In this

193

way other consultant colleagues can be introduced to management and from among them a natural successor to the clinical director should arise.

Subdirectorates should be appropriate to the size of the organisation and depend on the willingness and ability of a clinician to take the lead and the budgetary responsibility. Some clinicians would like the authority without the budgetary responsibility, but this is not workable and no subdirectorate should be set up under these circumstances. By introducing new consultants to the concept, and by ensuring that no purchase by the directorate can go ahead without money have been made available for it in the business plan, colleagues become drawn into the new style of management. There is often confusion in clinicians' minds between changes resulting from resource management, or audit and the audit cycle, or risk management, or standards of care, and inevitably the clinical director is blamed for them all.

Medical management

Staffing issues are critical; it is necessary to build in sufficient staff to cover emergencies as well as the contracted elective work with adequate provision for all areas and for training.

Flexible working patterns for senior medical staff and staff grades to relieve junior doctors' hours in "the new deal," have altered patterns of work and have made review of the way consultants and other medical staff work within the directorate an important part of annual planning. Fixed duties for life now seem unlikely for any new consultant staff.

Workload priorities require changes in traditional thinking. It is difficult to direct peers whose attitude is – as it has always been – to do their best for every patient with no thought of cost or consequences. The clinical director cannot commit colleagues to changes in workload or practice without consent, and can never over-ride the clinical judgement of colleagues.

To achieve success the clinical director needs the respect and confidence of colleagues. He or she must be supported in the directorate, though the clinical director is appointed not as a representative of a clinical group but to a post within the chief executive's management structure, and standards are set and performance appraised by a line manager, usually the chief executive.

194

Management of operating theatres is a critical factor in most anaesthetic directorates. In Basildon a consultant anaesthetist has been theatre manager since the introduction of general management in 1986 and it seemed natural that this should continue and that the theatre manager should become clinical director. The directorate now includes the rest of the anaesthetic department, intensive care, a new dedicated day unit with two integral theatres and 20 beds, and a pain clinic which is being developed since the recent appointment of a colleague with an interest. So, from running a relatively small area of the operating theatres, I became clinical director of a much larger area.

Given the fact that a doctor had been theatre manager, the nurses had become accustomed to the idea and were used to "their budget" for staff and theatre expenses being the responsibility of someone else. Given also that most expenditure on equipment in theatres is attributable to surgeons who are not accountable and who take no responsibility for the expense, nurse managers have been happy to offload that commitment.

Day unit

Setting up a new day unit has had a salutary effect. It has been possible to re-examine all practices in the operating theatres and wards and to provide a customer orientated, patient-focused service. A business plan stating the objectives and principles, setting standards, organising policies and procedures to achieve desired results, auditing and feeding back outcomes (both clinical and patient satisfaction) has been important. This style of management involves cooperation between medical staff, nursing staff, the audit clerk, and all other staff, as only together can best practice be achieved.

In a day unit with its integral theatre nursing staff can more easily be aware that their performance regulates the quality of the "product," the service and outcomes they provide for the customer – that is, the patient. Focusing on the patient rather than the tasks involved, motivating staff to think in a different way, and allowing them to try different ideas are powerful levers for change among nursing staff. The use of resources is crucial because without increased funding only greater productivity can improve the quality of service. In the day unit nurses can have close contact with the patients and can establish "named nurses" for patients, in line with the *Patients' charter*.[3]

Theatre efficiency

It has been possible to compare and contrast the style of the day unit with that in other areas such as operating theatre nurses visiting wards. The theatre nurses' time is a valuable resource and must be used in the most efficient way possible. Anaesthetists have time allocated in their contracts for visiting patients on the ward before operation. Should the unit pay for the time necessary for nurses to duplicate this for the sake of their professional status, morale, or education, and would this improve the service to patients? By allowing a pilot study, our theatre staff became convinced that this was not the best way, and instead have developed a patient information folder which seems to suit our patients and our nurses (both in theatre and on the wards), better than ward visiting.

Theatre efficiency has been under scrutiny for many years and the reports of the National Audit Office[4] and the Committee of Public Accounts (CPA), *The use of operating theatres in the NHS*, the Confidential Enquiry into Perioperative Deaths (CEPOD),[6] and the Bevan report,[7] all indicated that changes in the organisation of theatre services can improve both their use and standards of patient care. Bevan's proposal that a theatre services director should be appointed to establish and implement guidelines still holds good, as does the recommendation that the theatre services director should be either a doctor or someone well supported by a doctor. If the clinical director can undertake this role that is fine, or another clinician should be the head of a subdirectorate of theatres.

Some theatres are more efficient than others, some surgical teams more efficient than others. It is vitally important with contracting and even more so with the rapidly changing demands of general practitioner fundholders that efficiency is maximised. The efficiency of operating theatres and of anaesthetic departments has an important impact on surgical prices and therefore on contracts. In almost all theatres there are problems which can be dealt with at once to improve efficiency. Clear and agreed policies for throughput, case mix, length of lists, and so on, together with methods for monitoring these and enforcing the targets, are needed.

Theatre superintendents without clinical directors are at the mercy of surgeons who "own" their lists, who subject them to cancellations, to under-utilisation or over-running of lists, and who do not consult about changes in trends and in case mix (such as moves towards day surgery or the introduction of time-consuming minimally invasive surgery). Theatre superintendents need adequate support from their clinical directors as it is inappropriate to negotiate with an individual surgeon who may be the loudest shouter or greatest wheedler. Negotiations need to be between directorates and may involve a "theatre users group."

Non-medical theatre staff

The management of qualified, experienced, trained, non-medical staff in operating theatres requires constant review. We have been warned of fewer recruits to nursing; "Project 2000" means that student nurses will spend less time in theatre and the question remains as to whether they will want to work in operating theatres.[8]

The operating department practitioner (ODP) is now being trained to be a flexible multiskilled theatre worker with National Council for Vocational Qualification competence-based training. This will help but there will still be too few staff. The review of skills mix in the theatre is aimed at the recruitment, retention and turnover of staff, the changing patterns of service demand, value for money and cost control, and the desire to introduce flexible effective working patterns. A comprehensive review will help to understand and identify the options, and discussion on ways to resource the options can then follow.

This is no longer a nursing issue alone, but a directorate issue. Flexible use of staff may mean that the surgeon's scrub assistant is no longer the nurse, and the anaesthetist's assistant no longer the operating department assistant (ODA). Both will be ODPs working in a team environment where the skills of individual people will be effectively used, valued, and rewarded.

Qualifications called National Vocational Qualifications (NVQs) are being developed in all sectors of employment nationwide. The National Council for Vocational Qualifications accredits NVQs which meet its criteria. The requirements include: being based on national occupational standards relevant to employment; being unit based to allow for certification of unit credits and flexible training systems; and being assessed primarily at the workplace. NVQs are designed to benefit organisations, individual people, and the economy and are part of a government-led initiative to provide qualifications relating to work-based standards for a wider range of staff in vocational employment. The ODP "level 3" NVQ now equates with the old ODA qualification, but is almost certainly more relevant to the current needs of operating theatres. Nurses and ODPs can look forward to achieving NVQ additionally accredited units to cover more advanced competencies.

To support trained "level 3" staff or above, the "level 2" qualification is being introduced with some elements based on the Occupational Standard Council's units for health care workers together with some elements specific to operating departments.

Considerable investment of time and energy has been needed and will still be required to introduce the systems and train work-based assessors and local assessment coordinators for the NVQ units and this will have to be paid for.

There are anxieties that the introduction of level 2 ODP may encourage managers to reduce the skills mix in operating theatres, but clinical directors must ensure that adequate standards of skilled assistance for the anaesthetist and for the surgical and recovery teams are maintained.

The NVQ project for ODPs provides an alternative method of training and recognises the skills of appropriate staff who are working in the operating theatre. The twin hierarchies of nurse and ODA/ODP may become unified by a single pay spine in the near future, giving identical terms and conditions of service and rewarding skills gained.

Assessments of skills mix aim to make the best possible use of professional skills, but requirements will change as the contracts change and jobs for life are unlikely to be as unchangeable in the future as they have been previously. Continuous staff training and development will be needed to provide an adaptable multi-skilled and qualified workforce that can work flexibly to fulfil contracts.

Flexible working instead of "working to grade" will help to promote the extended role of the nurse and of the ODP and help towards the aims of *Achieving a balance* and *The new deal* for junior medical staff.[9 10]

Reviewing demarcation lines is important. New patterns of working have been pioneered by staff in the dedicated day unit with auxiliaries, porters, and nurses working flexibly and appropriately, preassessing and clerking patients and working with them as they go through the department. This has been developed not just because it gives value for money, but because it is definitely the best practice; best for staff in terms of morale, opportunities, and involvement, and best for patients in terms of quality, standards, and satisfaction. This approach has potential in other areas throughout the directorate. To achieve such change the role of the senior nurse manager who has a vision to maximise staff potential is crucial.

Budget management

If theatres and anaesthesia are combined, managing the budget will become more difficult. It is an expensive, high technology, labour-intensive directorate and almost inevitably there will be considerable pressures on its budget. Managing the budget in terms of medical staff and non medical staff, however complex, is simple compared with managing the rest of the budget for medical and surgical equipment, drugs, anaesthetic equipment, and equipment maintenance. Often the budget is dependent on use by others, on case mix, and on other innumerable variables. This, together with a complex system for ordering and supplying stores, can lead to many problems. Expensive items such as orthopaedic prostheses can be changed to the orthopaedic directorate together with an appropriate part of the budget to establish better management. In future effective mechanisms for making the people who use expensive items pay for them themselves will offer better control.

The budget of a directorate is derived from what was spent last year (a "rollover" or "historical" budget). Activity tends to control such a budget and identified items are often paid for if they are regarded as unavoidable. There is an attraction in the idea of selling services and having a bottom up or zero based budget. Given the poor quality of information and the difficulty of running an internal market with internal service agreements it may be better to stay with the "rollover" budget until clear advantage is gained from the change.

Staff health and safety

The clinical director has a duty of care towards staff in the directorate to see that they work in a safe environment. The issues involved include disposal of clinical and contaminated waste, lifting and handling equipment and patients, as well as Health and Safety Executive (Control of substances Hazardous to Health) Regulations, 1988, (COSHH) for handling harmful substances, use of radiation and lasers, and risks from using visual display units, and from needlestick injuries and infections (particularly hepatitis B and AIDS). Close liaison with the occupational health department to achieve targets is necessary and great care must be taken to look after staff. Hazard policies and procedures should be constantly reviewed. There is a duty of care to all grades from consultant colleagues to the greenest recruit and, to assist with this, induction days and the careful introduction of new and hazardous agents and techniques is essential. Allowance must be made for training and setting of standards when any new equipment or technique is introduced into the theatre.

Training for clinical directors

The clinical director attends the clinical directors' board which is the main operational management board in our structure. Here the clinical directors are not representatives of their directorates, but have a collective responsibility to maximise efficient use of resources and to ensure that performance is as specified in contracts throughout the hospital and within the budget. As a member of the directorate the individual will give expert opinion and may be called on to represent the services of colleagues and to ensure that financial constraints do not adversely affect quality in the directorate.

Training in management for clinical directors has taken various forms but some have been lucky enough to go to business schools funded by the Department of Health, or to be involved in action learning sets funded by the NHS Management Executive or other agencies. Inhouse management training in finance, personnel, and marketing has proved useful, as has training in business planning and negotiation skills. The investment in time and training is considerable and the hours of work required from a clinical director usually far exceed the contracted time negotiated for the post.

Conclusion

Resource management and the management of a clinical directorate are both about finding the right balance among quality, quantity, and cost, with audit as an essential tool to monitor the process. Anaesthetists want to see adherence to codes of practice and to professional standards. Even the most reluctant doctor nowadays has to recognise that all doctors work within budgets and must make the best use of resources available, mindful of the effect that any decision may have on the resources and choices available to others. There have always been decisions to make about access to medical care. There have always been inequalities. Colleagues have concerns about restrictions of access to health care for patients whose general practitioners are not fundholders and they are concerned that standards are being compromised. They are concerned also about being involved in a process which they do not like, and that they find irksome and distasteful. But however reluctant an individual anaesthetist is, most would agree that they must emphasise the importance of anaesthesia in modern medical care. They recognise anaesthesia as a core service and that some anaesthetists must be involved in planning anaesthesia, theatres, and related services including dealing with all the staff and the budgetary responsibilities. At present this is best done through the clinical directorate.

1 *Guidelines on duties of chairmen of divisions of anaesthesia.* London: Association of Anaesthetists of Great Britain and Ireland, 1988.
2 *NHS management changes – implications for anaesthetists.* London: Association of Anaesthetists of Great Britain and Ireland, 1992.
3 Department of Health. *The patient's charter.* London: HMSO, 1991.
4 Comptroller and Auditor General. *Use of NHS operating theatres in England: a progress report.* London: National Audit Office, 1991.
5 National Audit Office. *Use of operating theatres in the National Health Service.* London: HMSO, 1987.
6 Buck N, Devlin HB, Lunn JN. *Report of a confidential enquiry into perioperative deaths.* London: King's Fund and the Nuffield Provincial Hospitals Trust, 1987.
7 NHS Management Executive. The Management and Utilisation of Operating Departments. London: HMSO, 1989. (Chairman PG Bevan).
8 *Project 2000. A new preparation for practice.* London: United Kingdom Central Council for Nursing Midwifery and Health Visiting, 1986.
9 *Hospital Medical Staff: Achieving a balance.* Plan for action in brief. London: DHSS, 1988.
10 NHS Management Executive. *Junior doctors: The new deal.* London: NHSME, 1991.

Index